NUTRITION SUPPORT MANUAL

First-Time Teaching Tips and Visual Lecture Outlines

for

Nutrition: An Applied Approach

Second Edition

Janice Thompson, Ph.D., FACSM
UNIVERSITY OF BRISTOL
UNIVERSITY OF NEW MEXICO

Melinda Manore, Ph.D., RD, FACSM
OREGON STATE UNIVERSITY

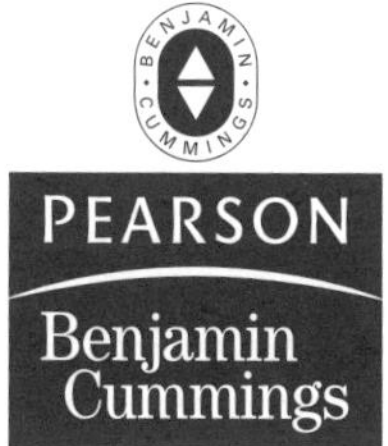

San Francisco Boston New York
Cape Town Hong Kong London Madrid Mexico City
Montreal Munich Paris Singapore Sydney Tokyo Toronto

Acquisitions Editor: Sandra Lindelof
Development Manager: Claire Alexander
Senior Project Editor: Marie Beaugureau
Editorial Assistant: Jacob Evans
Managing Editor: Deborah Cogan
Production Supervisor: Mary O'Connell
Manufacturing Buyer: Dorothy Cox
Marketing Manager: Neena Bali
Cover Photograph: StockFood Munich/Stockfood
Supplement Cover Designer: 17th Street Studios
Main Text Cover Designer: Jeanne Calabrese
Design and Composition: PrePress PMG

ISBN-10 0-321-53651-7
ISBN-13 978-0-321-53651-8

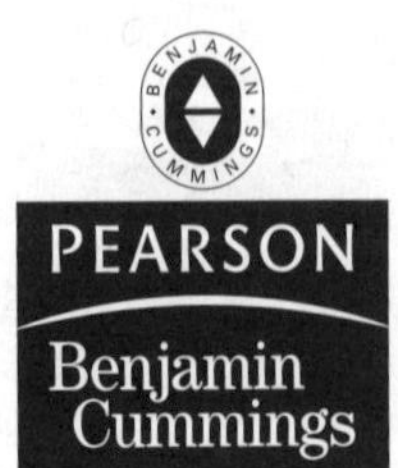

1 2 3 4 5 6 7 8—MAL— 12 11 10 09 08
www.aw-bc.com

How to Use this Manual

Preparing for a course can often be the most daunting part of teaching it! This manual can help anyone teaching the nutrition course prepare lectures, activities, and syllabi, but it was especially focused for teachers who are preparing and creating their introductory nutrition lecture materials for the first time. Each section of the manual offers advice and instruction on how to:

- organize the content throughout the course,
- prepare clear and informative materials in the least amount of time,
- and provide the best interactive learning experience for your students.

The Visual Lecture Outlines in **Part 1** will help you prepare PowerPoint or Transparency Acetate lectures. All of the images, animations, PPT slides, and videos listed are available on our Instructor's Media Manager. In addition, the lecture outlines will point out what key terms should be covered, which interactive activities to introduce throughout your lecture, and what testing material is appropriate after covering the content. General best practices for teaching are covered in **Part 2**, and **Part 3** will show you how to incorporate our diet analysis software, MyDietAnalysis, into your course. The Tips for Using MyNutritionLab, offered in **Part 4**, is a valuable resource for any instructors with online components to their courses. The sample syllabi in **Part 5**, will show you examples of how to organize your lectures given inevitable time constraints, and **Part 6** provides you with the full set of our popular *Great Ideas in Teaching Nutrition* newsletters, which have helped many professors add fun interactive activities to their classrooms.

Acknowledgements

Thank you to Bassam M. Salameh, California State University, Bakersfield, and James Bailey, University of Tennessee, Knoxville, for providing the samples of the 12- and 16-week syllabi in Part 5. Many thanks to Barbara Hewitt, M.S., from Diablo Valley College for creating the original content from which the MyNutritionLab Primer in Part 4 was created. Finally, our gratitude goes out to Linda Fleming, Middlesex Community College, who wrote the ABC News Video Discussion Questions and the Nutrition Debate and MyDietAnalysis activities.

Contents

Part 1: Visual Lecture Outlines

Chapter 1:	The Role of Nutrition in Our Health	1
Chapter 2:	Designing a Healthful Diet	5
Chapter 3:	The Human Body: Are We Really What We Eat?	9
Chapter 4:	Carbohydrates: Plant-Derived Energy Nutrients	15
	In Depth: Alcohol	21
Chapter 5:	Fat: An Essential Energy-Supplying Nutrient	25
Chapter 6:	Proteins: Crucial Components of All Body Tissues	31
	In Depth: Vitamins and Minerals: Micronutrients with Macro Powers	37
Chapter 7:	Nutrients Involved in Fluid and Electrolyte Balance	41
Chapter 8:	Nutrients Involved in Antioxidant Function	47
	In Depth: Phytochemicals and Functional Foods	51
Chapter 9:	Nutrients Involved in Bone Health	53
Chapter 10:	Nutrients Involved in Energy Metabolism and Blood Health	59
Chapter 11:	Achieving and Maintaining a Healthful Body Weight	63
Chapter 12:	Nutrition and Physical Activity: Keys to Good Health	69
Chapter 13:	Disordered Eating	73
Chapter 14:	Food Safety and Technology: Impact on Consumers	79
Chapter 15:	Nutrition Through the Lifecycle: Pregnancy and the First Year of Life	85
Chapter 16:	Nutrition Through the Lifecycle: Childhood to Late Adulthood	89
	In Depth: Global Nutrition	93

Part 2: Teaching Tips for First-Time Instructors and Adjunct Professors **97**

Part 3: Teaching Tips for MyDietAnalysis 105

Part 4: Tips for Using MyNutritionLab 113

Part 5: Sample Syllabi for Introductory Nutrition

Sample Syllabus for Introduction to Nutrition: 12-week Course 119

Sample Syllabus for Introduction to Nutrition: 16-week Course 122

Part 6: Great Ideas!

Great Ideas in Teaching Nutrition, Volume 1 127

Great Ideas in Teaching Nutrition, Volume 2 135

The Role of Nutrition in Our Health

1

Chapter at a Glance

I. What Is Nutrition?
II. Why Is Nutrition Important?
III. What Are Nutrients?
IV. How Can I Figure Out My Nutrient Needs?
V. Research Study Results: Who Can We Believe?
VI. Nutrition Advice: Who Can You Trust?

Visual Lecture Outline

I. What Is Nutrition? (p. 4)

Instructor Tools: Chapter 1 PPT slides, Chapter 1 PRS Clicker Questions slide 1

II. Why Is Nutrition Important? (p. 4)

a. Nutrition Is One of Several Factors Contributing to Wellness
b. A Healthful Diet Can Prevent Some Diseases and Reduce Your Risk for Others

Key Terms: nutrition, wellness

Instructor Tools: Chapter 1 PPT slides, TAs 1–3, 12

Images:

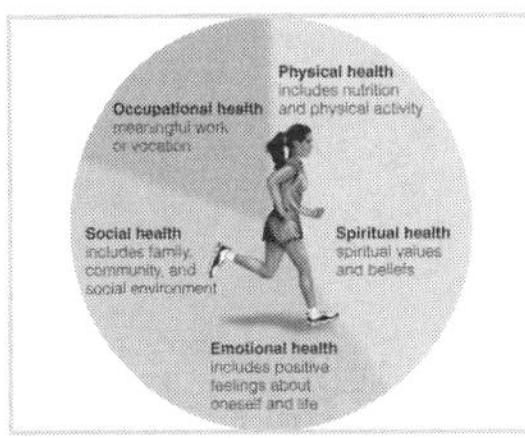

Figure 1.1
Many factors contribute to an individual's wellness.

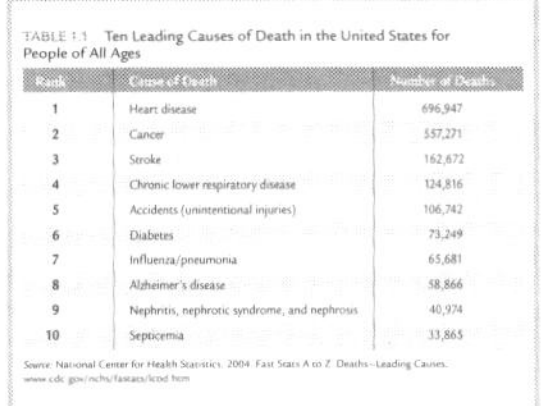

TABLE 1.1 Ten Leading Causes of Death in the United States for People of All Ages

Rank	Cause of Death	Number of Deaths
1	Heart disease	696,947
2	Cancer	557,271
3	Stroke	162,672
4	Chronic lower respiratory disease	124,816
5	Accidents (unintentional injuries)	106,742
6	Diabetes	73,249
7	Influenza/pneumonia	65,681
8	Alzheimer's disease	58,866
9	Nephritis, nephrotic syndrome, and nephrosis	40,974
10	Septicemia	33,865

Source: National Center for Health Statistics. 2004. Fast Stats A to Z. Deaths–Leading Causes. www.cdc.gov/nchs/fastats/lcod.htm

Table 1.1
Ten Leading Causes of Death in the United States for People of All Ages

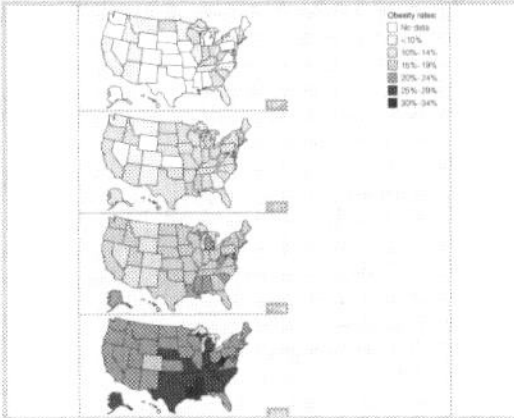

Figure 1.2
Obesity rates across the United States from 1985 to 2005.

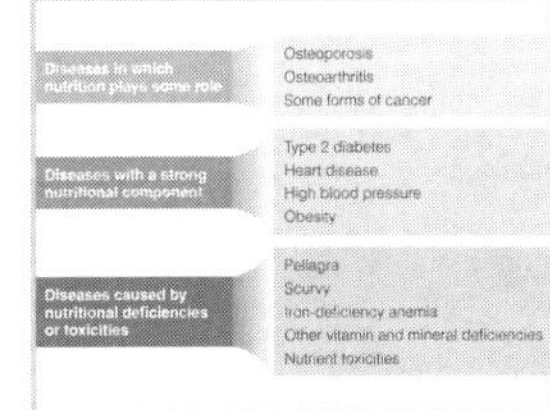

Figure 1.3
The relationship between nutrition and human disease.

III. What Are Nutrients? (p. 6)

a. Carbohydrates, Fats, and Proteins Are Nutrients That Provide Energy
b. Vitamins Assist in the Regulation of Biological Processes
c. Minerals Assist in the Regulation of Many Body Functions
d. Water Supports All Body Functions

Key Terms: nutrients, organic, inorganic, macronutrients, carbohydrates, fats, proteins, vitamins, metabolism, micronutrients, fat-soluble vitamins, water-soluble vitamins, minerals, major minerals, trace minerals

Instructor Tools: Chapter 1 PPT slides, Chapter 1 PRS Clicker Questions slides 2–3, TAs 4–7, 13–14

Images:

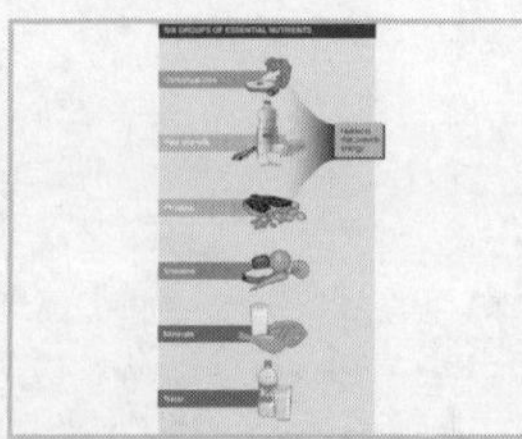

Figure 1.4
The six groups of essential nutrients found in the foods we consume.

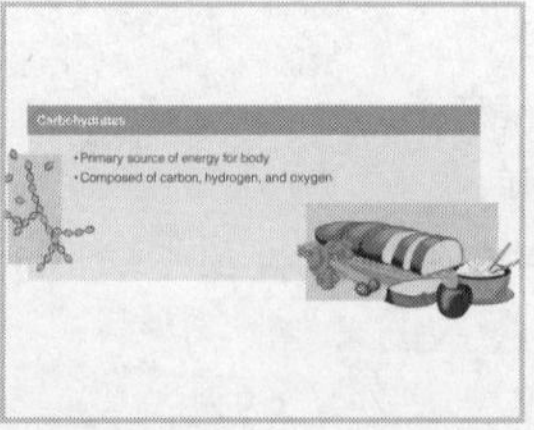

Figure 1.5
Carbohydrates are a primary source of energy for our bodies and are found in a wide variety of foods.

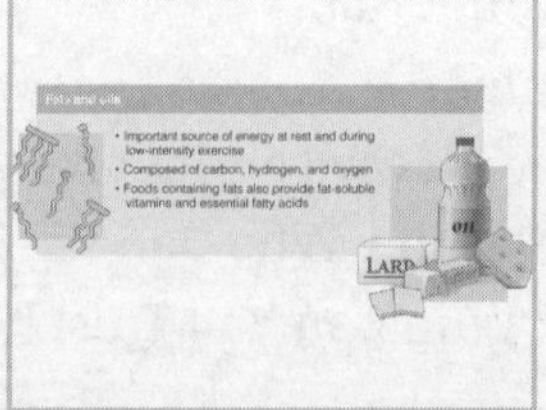

Figure 1.6
Fats are an important energy source during rest and low-intensity exercise.

• Support tissue growth, repair, and maintenance
• Composed of carbon, hydrogen, oxygen, and nitrogen

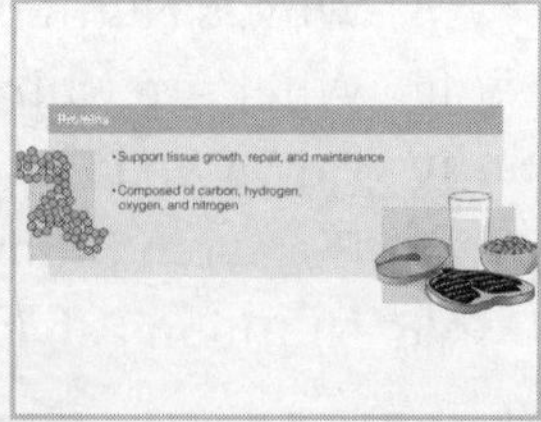

Figure 1.7
Proteins contain nitrogen in addition to carbon, hydrogen, and oxygen.

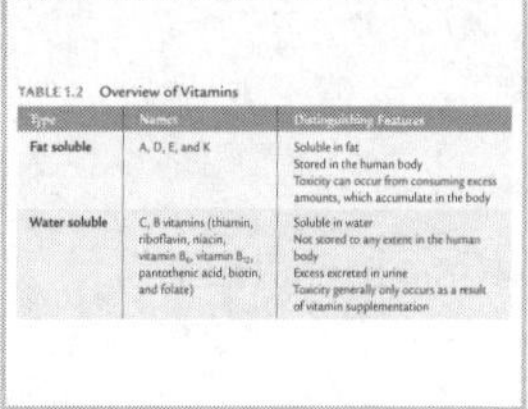

TABLE 1.2 Overview of Vitamins

Type	Names	Distinguishing Features
Fat soluble	A, D, E, and K	Soluble in fat Stored in the human body Toxicity can occur from consuming excess amounts, which accumulate in the body
Water soluble	C, B vitamins (thiamin, riboflavin, niacin, vitamin B_6, vitamin B_{12}, pantothenic acid, biotin, and folate)	Soluble in water Not stored to any extent in the human body Excess excreted in urine Toxicity generally only occurs as a result of vitamin supplementation

Table 1.2
Overview of Vitamins

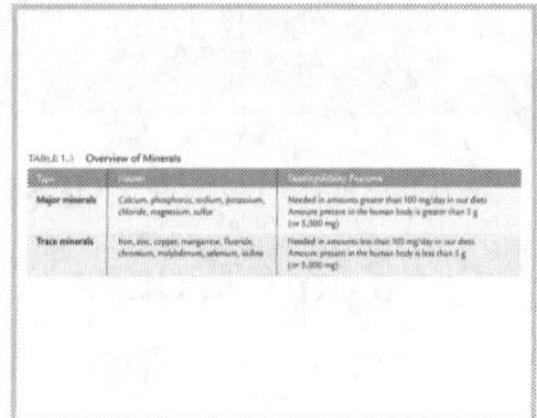

TABLE 1.3 Overview of Minerals

Type	Names	Distinguishing Features
Major minerals	Calcium, phosphorus, sodium, potassium, chloride, magnesium, sulfur	Needed in amounts greater than 100 mg/day in our diets Amount present in the human body is greater than 5 g (or 5,000 mg)
Trace minerals	Iron, zinc, copper, manganese, fluoride, chromium, molybdenum, selenium, iodine	Needed in amounts less than 100 mg/day in our diets Amount present in the human body is less than 5 g (or 5,000 mg)

Table 1.3
Overview of Minerals

IV. How Can I Figure Out My Nutrient Needs? (p. 13)

a. Use the Dietary Reference Intakes to Check Your Nutrient Intake
b. Calculating Your Unique Nutrient Needs

Key Terms: Dietary Reference Intakes (DRIs), Estimated Average Requirement (EAR), Recommended Dietary Allowance (RDA), Adequate Intake (AI), Tolerable Upper Intake Level (UL), Estimated Energy Requirement (EER), Acceptable Macronutrient Distribution Range (AMDR)

Instructor Tools: Chapter 1 PPT slides, Chapter 1 PRS Clicker Questions slides 4–5, TAs 8–10, 15

Animation: *DRI Determination*

Images:

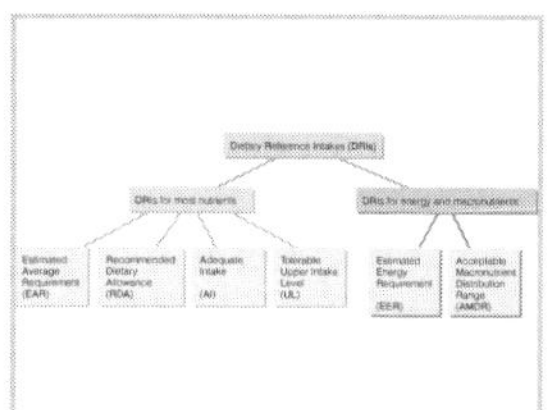

Figure 1.8
The Dietary Reference Intakes (DRIs) for all nutrients.

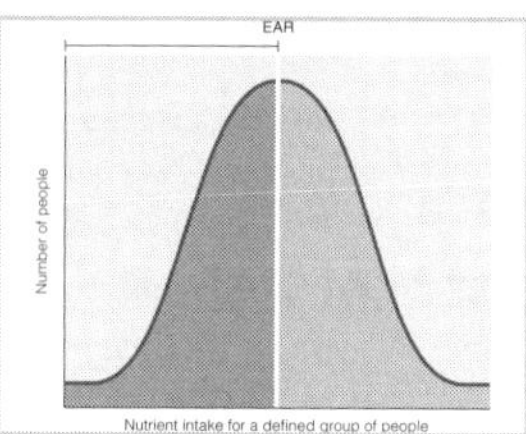

Figure 1.9
The Estimated Average Requirement (EAR).

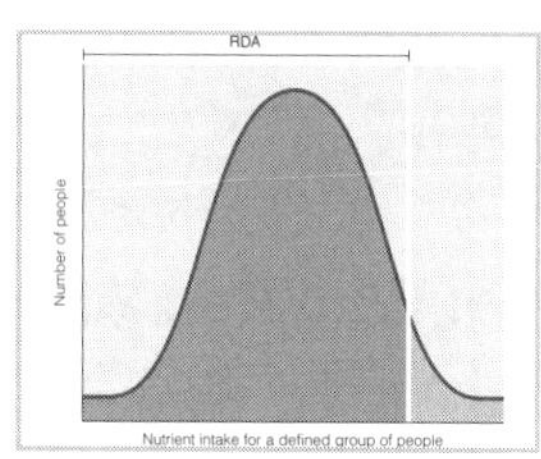

Figure 1.10
The Recommended Dietary Allowance (RDA).

TABLE 1.4 Acceptable Macronutrient Distribution Ranges (AMDRs) for Healthful Diets

Nutrient	AMDR*
Carbohydrate	45–65%
Fat	20–35%
Protein	10–35%

*AMDR values are expressed as percent of total energy or as percent of total calories.
Source: Institute of Medicine, Food and Nutrition Board. 2005. *Dietary Reference Intakes for Energy, Carbohydrates, Fiber, Fat, Fatty Acids, Cholesterol, Protein, and Amino Acids (Macronutrients).* Washington, DC: National Academies Press. Reprinted by permission.

Table 1.4
Acceptable Macronutrient Distribution Ranges (AMDR) for Healthful Diets

Activities:

1. Estimate portion sizes of premeasured foods that have been placed in the classroom. Examples of foods that can be used for this activity include salad or vegetables, sliced fruit, cereal, cooked meat, snack foods such as potato chips, popcorn, or nuts, butter or peanut butter, cheese, and pasta or rice. Ask students to make note of the most appropriate units for measuring these foods. For example, note differences between fluid ounces versus solid ounces and weight versus volume.
2. Have students bring to class a food product that contains a Nutrition Facts label, and instruct them to examine their labels and those of their classmates in small groups. Ask them to note the following:
   a. Which of the six nutrient classes are represented on the labels?
   b. Are any nutrient classes missing from the labels?
   c. Is the information complete for each nutrient class?
   d. Why might information about some nutrients be missing?

V. Research Study Results: Who Can We Believe? (p. 17)

a. Research Involves Applying the Scientific Method
b. Various Types of Research Studies Tell Us Different Stories
c. Use Your Knowledge of Research to Help You Evaluate Media Reports

Key Terms: hypothesis, theory

Instructor Tools: Chapter 1 PPT slides, TA 11

Image:

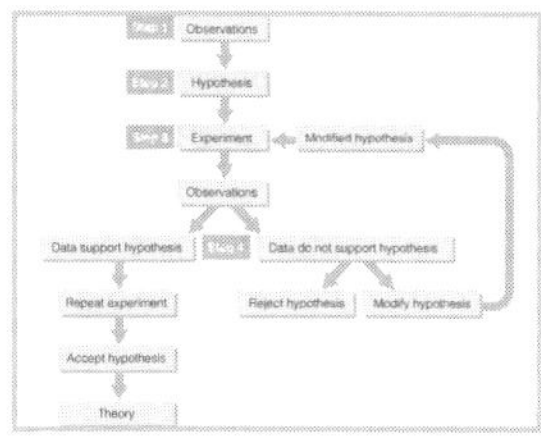

Figure 1.11
The scientific method.

Activity:

List the steps of the scientific method in the wrong order. Ask the class to place them, one by one, in the correct order.

VI. Nutrition Advice: Who Can You Trust? (p. 24)

a. Trustworthy Experts Are Educated and Credentialed

b. Government Sources of Information Are Usually Trustworthy

c. Professional Organizations Provide Reliable Nutrition Information

Key Terms: Centers for Disease Control and Prevention (CDC), National Health and Nutrition Examination Survey (NHANES), 24-hour recall, Behavioral Risk Factor Surveillance System (BRFSS), National Institutes of Health (NIH)

Instructor Tools: Chapter 1 PPT slides

Activities:

1. Log on to the Tufts University Nutrition Navigator Web site at http://navigator.tufts.edu. The purpose of this site is to identify reliable sources of nutrition information. Have students search for information on a topic that interests them such as heart disease, folic acid, iron, etc. They can then report to the class on their findings.
2. Invite one or more guest speakers who work in the area of nutrition to share their job experiences with the class.

VII. Additional Chapter 1 Instructor Tools

MyDietAnalysis Activity: Have your students choose three days during which their eating habits are typical. A good guideline is to include two week days and one weekend day. Have them record all foods and drinks they consume for each of the three days. Be sure they estimate the quantities of each item to the best of their abilities. Ask them to enter this information into their diet analysis software and to compare their intakes to the DRIs appropriate for their age and gender. It is not necessary to meet 100% of each DRI every day. A general guideline is meeting between 80% and 120% of the requirements over a one-week period. Have them answer the following questions:

1. For how many nutrients analyzed did you meet requirements?
2. How many nutrients were less than 80% of requirements?
3. How many nutrients were greater than 120% of requirements?
4. Keep this assessment for use in future activities.

Nutrition Debate Activity: To demonstrate an easily observable genetic trait, distribute PTC tasting paper to your students. Compare the number of tasters to non-tasters in the class.

Printed TestBank: Pages 1–13 (TestGen Chapter 1)

Quiz Show PowerPoints: Chapter 1

Lecture Teaching Tips CD: Why We Wrote the Book, New For This Edition, and Introduction to the Book (for Students)

Designing a Healthful Diet

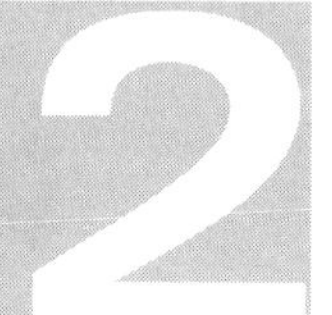

Chapter at a Glance

I. What Is a Healthful Diet?
II. What Tools Can Help Me Design a Healthful Diet?
III. Can Eating Out Be Part of a Healthful Diet?

Visual Lecture Outline

I. What Is a Healthful Diet? (p. 38)

a. A Healthful Diet Is Adequate
b. A Healthful Diet Is Moderate
c. A Healthful Diet Is Balanced
d. A Healthful Diet Is Varied

Key Terms: healthful diet, adequate diet, moderation, balanced diet, variety

Instructor Tools: Chapter 2 PPT slides, Chapter 2 PRS Clicker Questions slide 1

II. What Tools Can Help Me Design a Healthful Diet? (p. 40)

a. Food Labels
b. Dietary Guidelines for Americans
c. MyPyramid: The Food Guide Pyramid
d. Eating Plans

abc NEWS **Lecture Launcher Video:**

Food Labels and Portion Size

abc NEWS **Video Discussion Questions:**

1. What do food labels have to offer in diet planning?
2. Do food labels accurately reflect the portions most people eat?
3. How could food labels be revised to be more useful to the consumer?

Key Terms: Nutrition Facts Panel, percent Daily Values (%DV), Dietary Guidelines for Americans, MyPyramid, discretionary calories, ounce-equivalent, nutrient density, DASH diet, Exchange System

Instructor Tools: Chapter 2 PPT slides, Chapter 2 PRS Clicker Questions slides 2–5, TAs 16–45

Animation: *Reading Labels*

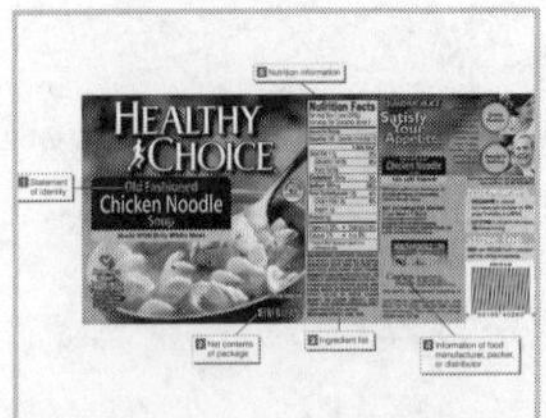
Figure 2.1
The five primary components that are required for food labels.

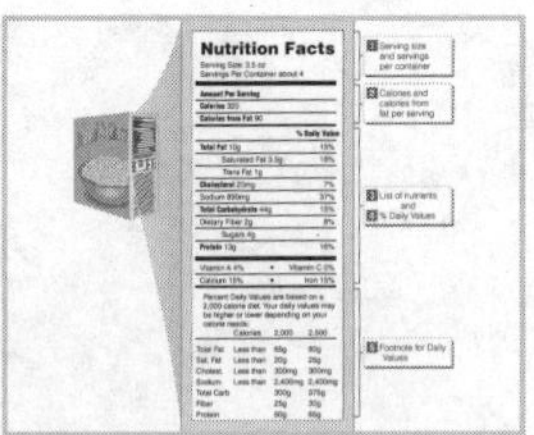
Figure 2.2
The Nutrition Facts Panel.

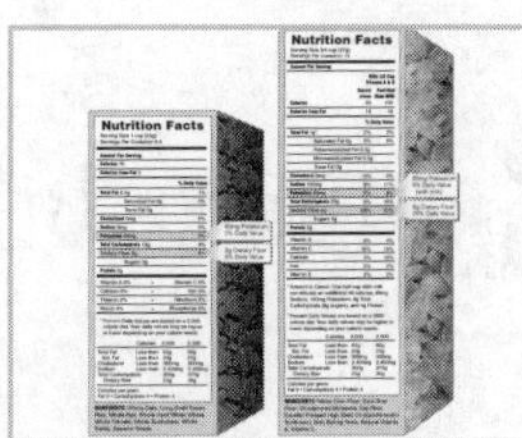
Figure 2.3
Labels from two breakfast cereals.

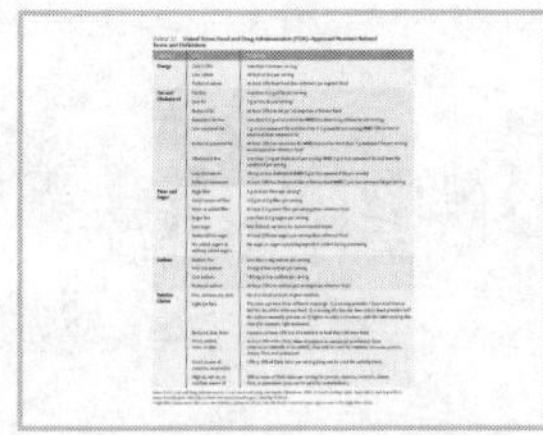
Table 2.1
FDA Approved Nutrient-Related Terms and Definitions

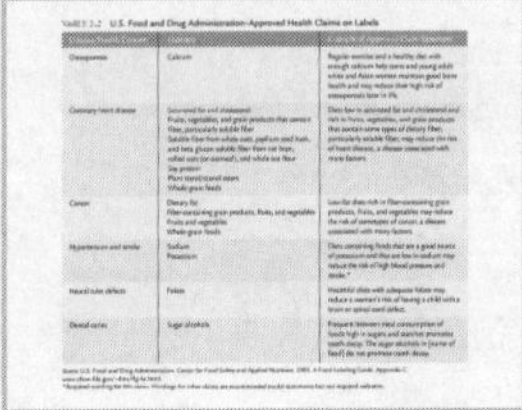
Table 2.2
FDA Approved Health Claims on Labels

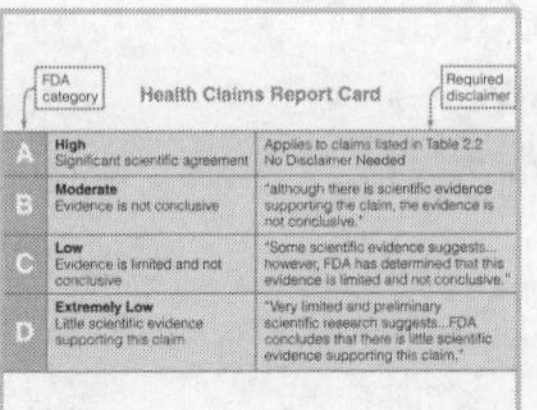
Figure 2.4
The FDA's Health Claims Report Card.

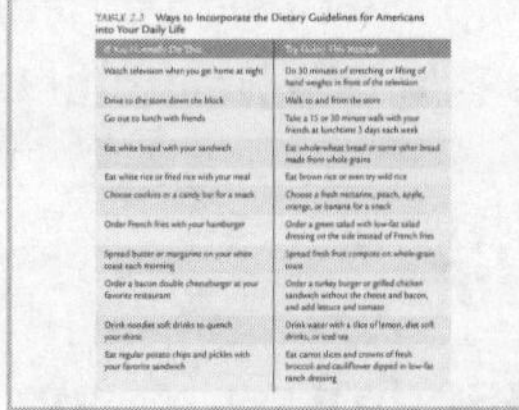
Table 2.3
Ways to Incorporate the Dietary Guidelines for Americans into Your Daily Life

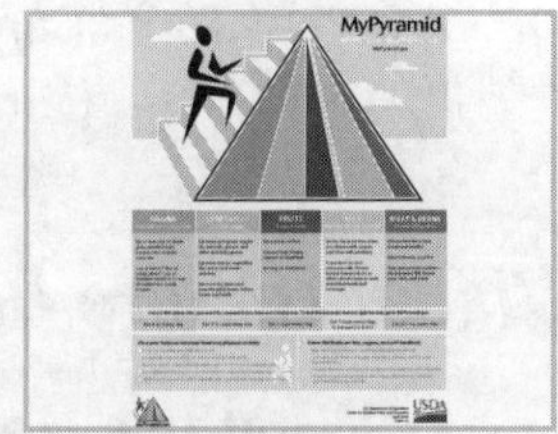
Figure 2.5
The USDA MyPyramid.

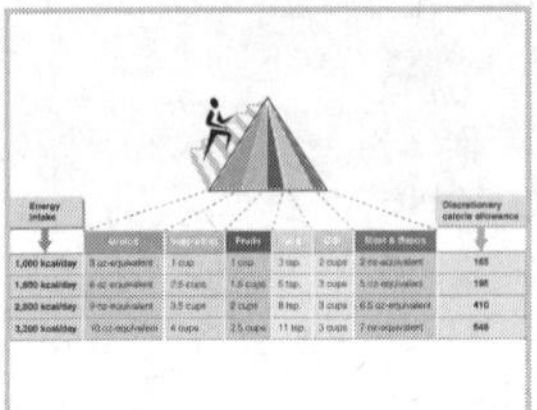
Figure 2.6
Sample diets from MyPyramid at four different energy intakes.

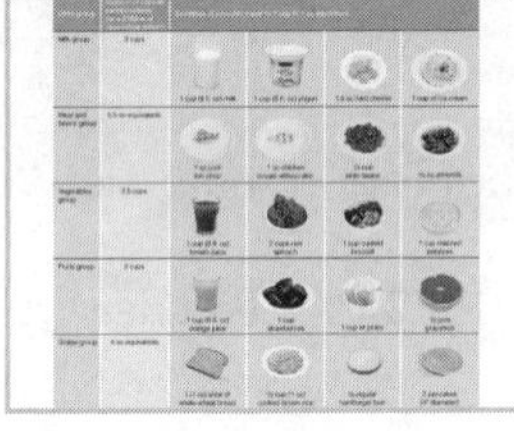
Figure 2.7
Examples of serving sizes for foods in each food group of MyPyramid for a 2,000 kcal food intake pattern.

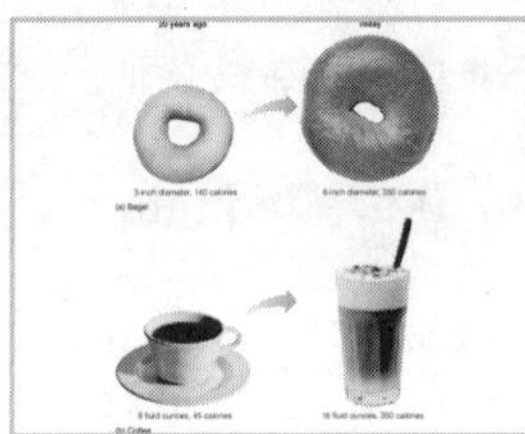
Figure 2.8
Examples of increases in food portion sizes over the past 20 years.

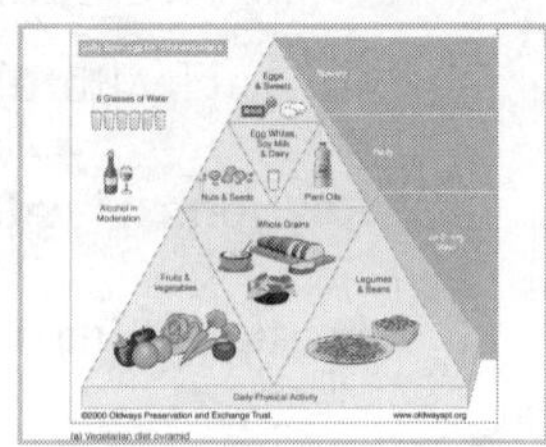
Figure 2.9a
The Vegetarian Diet Pyramid

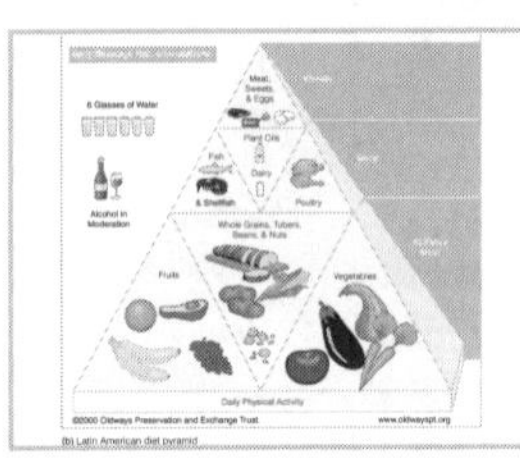
Figure 2.9b
The Latin American Diet Pyramid.

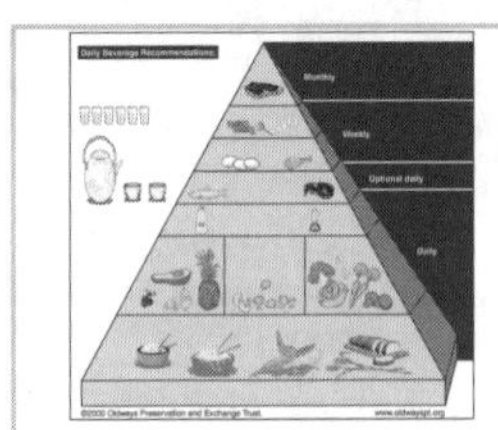
Figure 2.9c
The Asian Diet Pyramid.

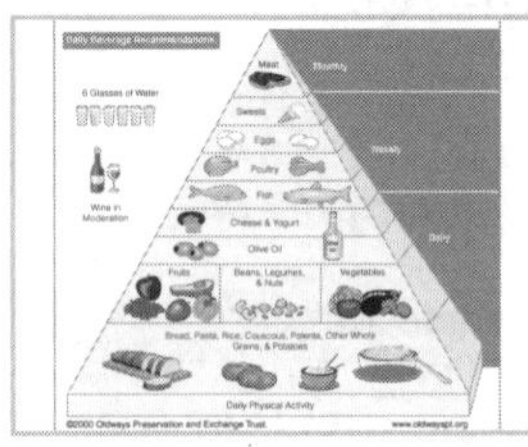
Figure 2.10
The Mediterranean Diet Pyramid.

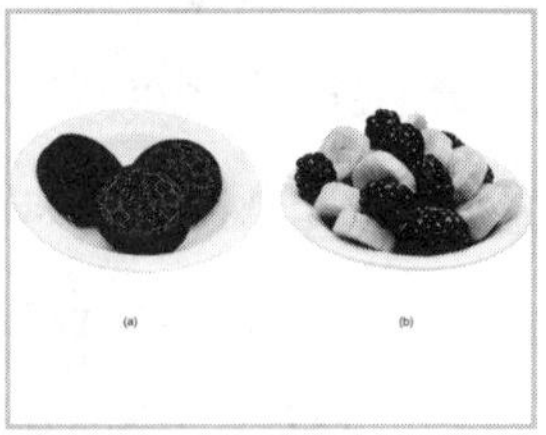
Figure 2.11
Examples of foods that are low or high in nutrient density.

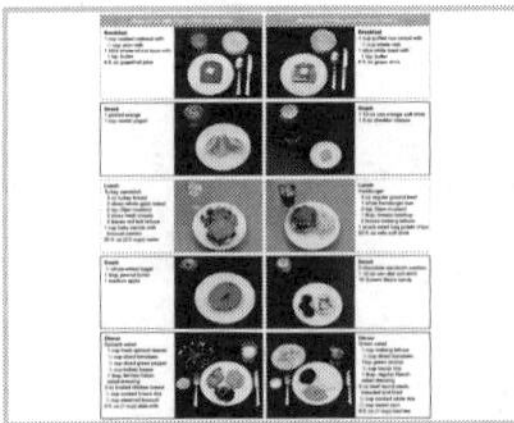
Figure 2.12
High nutrient density vs. low nutrient density meals.

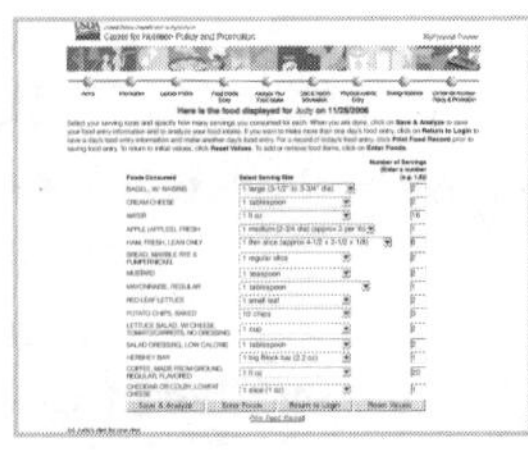
Figure 2.13a
Analysis of one day of Judy's diet using MyPyramid Tracker.

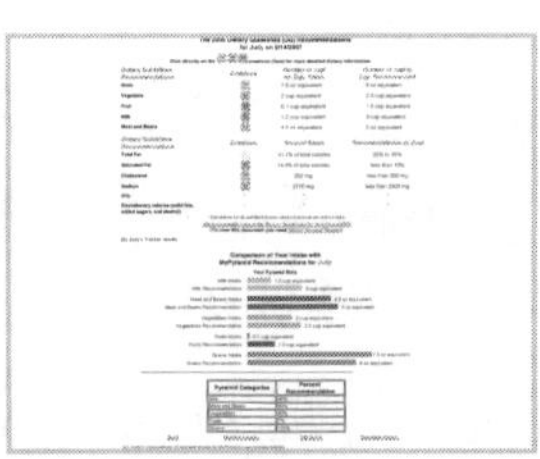
Figure 2.13b

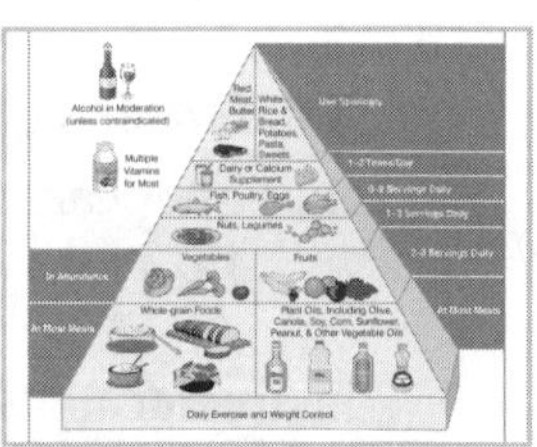
Figure 2.14
The Healthy Eating Pyramid.

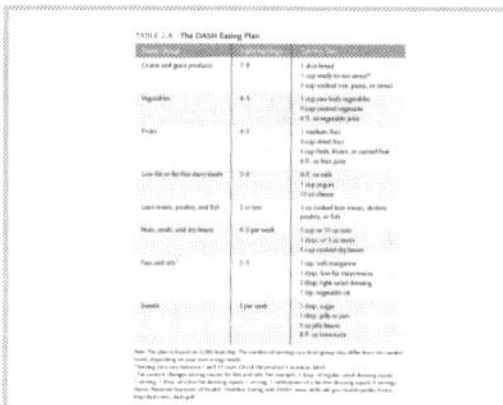
Table 2.4
The DASH Eating Plan

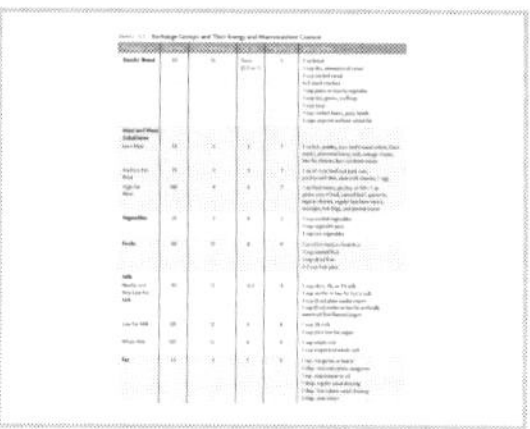
Table 2.5
Exchange Groups and Their Energy and Macronutrient Content.

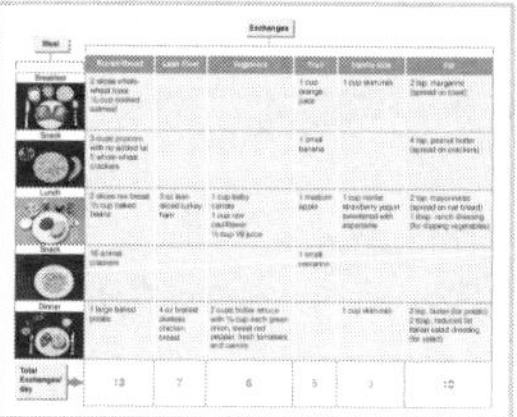
Figure 2.15
Example of a one-day meal plan for a 2,600 calorie diet using the Exchange System.

Activities:

1. Students should use the food intake journal they previously completed to determine whether or not their intake conforms to the Dietary Guidelines. Refer to the inside front cover of the text for a summary of the Guidelines. Students should answer the following questions:
   a. How many Dietary Guidelines do you meet?
   b. How might you change your diet or lifestyle to more closely meet recommendations?
2. Have students bring to class three food products that contain a food label. Instruct them to examine and discuss the ingredients list and the Nutrition Facts Panel in small groups. Have them answer the following questions for each label:
   a. What is the ingredient present in the largest amount?
   b. What is the serving size for the product?
   c. Is the stated serving size the amount you would normally eat?
   d. What is the number of calories per serving?
   e. What is the amount of fat (in grams) per serving?
   f. For each food product, discuss whether this would be considered a nutrient-dense food. Students should give reasons for their answer.
3. Have an "international feast" with groups of students using the variations of the previous USDA Food Guide Pyramid to plan the meals. Variations discussed in the text include the Vegetarian Diet Pyramid, African American Diet Pyramid, Latin American Diet Pyramid, Asian Diet Pyramid, and Mediterranean Diet Pyramid.

III. Can Eating Out Be Part of a Healthful Diet? (p. 71)

a. The Hidden Costs of Eating Out
b. The Healthful Way to Eat Out

abc NEWS **Lecture Launcher Video:**

Diet Meals

abc NEWS **Video Discussion Questions:**

1. Would you choose a meal specifically because it is identified as a "healthy" choice? Why or why not?
2. Are the meals identified in some chain restaurants as healthier choices actually healthy? Explain.

3. What questions are reasonable to ask to find out if a meal is actually healthy?
4. Do you think all restaurants should be required to list nutrition facts on their menus? Why or why not?

Instructor Tools: Chapter 2 PPT slides, TAs 46–47

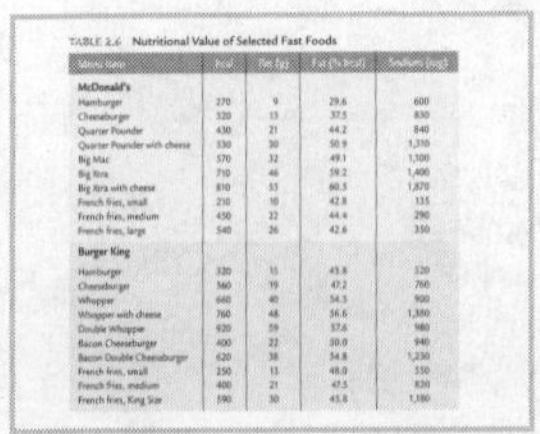

TABLE 2.6 Nutritional Value of Selected Fast Foods

[illegible]	[illegible]	[illegible]	[illegible]	[illegible]
McDonald's				
Hamburger	270	9	29.6	600
Cheeseburger	320	13	37.5	830
Quarter Pounder	430	21	44.2	840
Quarter Pounder with cheese	530	30	50.9	1,310
Big Mac	570	32	49.1	1,100
Big Xtra	710	46	59.2	1,400
Big Xtra with cheese	810	55	60.5	1,870
French fries, small	210	10	42.8	135
French fries, medium	450	22	44.4	290
French fries, large	540	26	42.6	350
Burger King				
Hamburger	320	15	43.8	520
Cheeseburger	360	19	47.2	760
Whopper	660	40	54.5	900
Whopper with cheese	760	48	56.6	1,380
Double Whopper	920	59	57.6	980
Bacon Cheeseburger	400	22	50.0	940
Bacon Double Cheeseburger	620	38	54.8	1,230
French fries, small	250	13	48.0	550
French fries, medium	400	21	47.5	820
French fries, King Size	590	30	45.8	1,180

Table 2.6
Nutritional Value of Selected Fast Foods

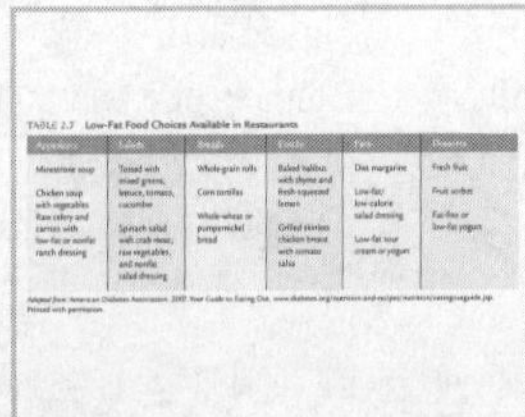

TABLE 2.7 Low-Fat Food Choices Available in Restaurants

[illegible]	[illegible]	[illegible]	[illegible]	[illegible]	[illegible]
Minestrone soup	Tossed with mixed greens, lettuce, tomato, cucumber	Whole-grain rolls	Baked halibut with thyme and fresh-squeezed lemon	Diet margarine	Fresh fruit
Chicken soup with vegetables	Spinach salad with crab meat, raw vegetables, and nonfat salad dressing	Corn tortillas	Grilled skinless chicken breast with tomato salsa	Low-fat/low-calorie salad dressing	Fruit sorbet
Raw celery and carrots with low-fat or nonfat ranch dressing		Whole-wheat or pumpernickel bread		Low-fat sour cream or yogurt	Fat-free or low-fat yogurt

[illegible]

Table 2.7
Low-fat Food Choices Available in Restaurants

Activity:

Have students visit a restaurant that provides nutrition facts for its meals. As an alternative, this information can be accessed online for many restaurants. Students should try to plan a healthful meal from the restaurant's menu. Discussion in class can address whether or not it was possible to find healthy options. Students should also state if they would order the healthy option if they were eating at this restaurant. Why or why not?

IV. Additional Chapter 2 Instructor Tools

MyDietAnalysis Activity: Using the nutritional assessment previously completed, students should note the MyPyramid information provided by their diet analysis software and answer the following questions:

a. Do your intakes meet recommendations for each food group?
b. What food groups are you high in?
c. What food groups are you low in?
d. What changes can you make in your diet to more closely meet the recommendations of MyPyramid?

Nutrition Debate Activity: MyPyramid is the most recent attempt by the USDA to promote a healthy diet and lifestyle. Although it has addressed some criticisms of the previous Food Guide Pyramid, experts have already expressed concerns about this newest version, as well. Instruct students to read the Nutrition Debate carefully and make note of the improvements and the concerns surrounding MyPyramid. Then, working in small groups, ask students to design a food guide of their own that they believe can improve on the current version. Have each group present their food guide to the class.

Printed TestBank: Pages 14–27 (TestGen Chapter 2)

MyDietAnalysis Online Assignments: Judy: Selecting a Perfect Diet; Theo: An Athlete

Quiz Show PowerPoints: Chapter 2

The Human Body: Are We Really What We Eat?

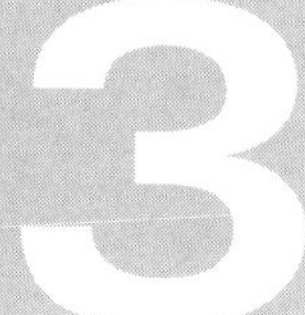

Chapter at a Glance

I. Why Do We Want to Eat What We Want to Eat?
II. Are We Really What We Eat?
III. What Happens to the Food We Eat?
IV. How Does the Body Coordinate and Regulate Digestion?
V. What Disorders Are Related to Digestion, Absorption, and Elimination?

Visual Lecture Outline

I. Why Do We Want to Eat What We Want to Eat? (p. 82)

a. The Hypothalamus Prompts Hunger in Response to Various Signals

b. Environmental Cues Trigger Appetite

abc NEWS **Lecture Launcher Video:**

Meal Replacements

abc NEWS **Video Discussion Questions:**

1. Do you think meal replacements have a place in a healthy diet? Why or why not?
2. What are some of the drawbacks of meal replacement products?
3. What are some of the benefits of meal replacement products?
4. Do you think meal replacement products aid in weight loss? Why or why not?

Key Terms: hunger, appetite, anorexia, hypothalamus, hormone

Instructor Tools: Chapter 3 PPT slides, Chapter 3 PRS Clicker Questions slide 1, TAs 48–49

Animation: *Control of Appetite: Hunger and Satiety*

Images:

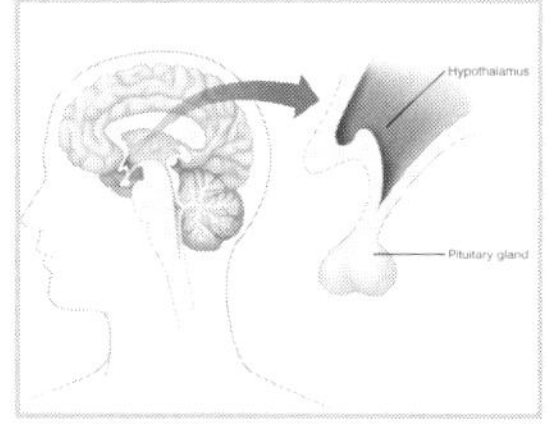

Figure 3.1
The hypothalamus triggers hunger by integrating signals from nerve cells throughout the body as well as from messages carried by hormones.

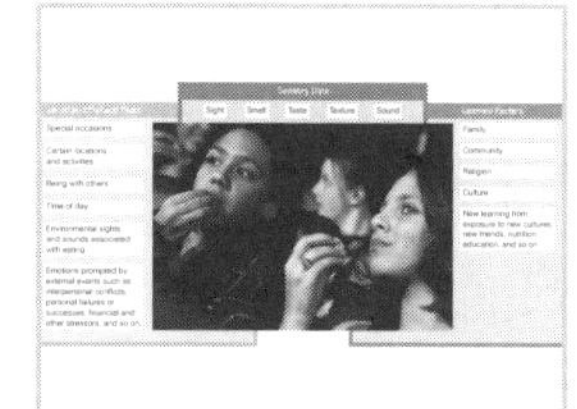

Figure 3.2
Appetite is a drive to consume specific foods, such as popcorn at the movies.

Activity:

Have students work in small groups to demonstrate the connection between taste, smell, and food texture. Bring small samples of various foods to class. Each student in the group can take a turn tasting a food item using no other senses. To do this, the student taster should close his or her eyes and pinch nostrils closed. Another student in the group should gently place the food on the taster's tongue. The taster should try to identify the food without chewing or moving the food in the mouth. The taster should then chew the food to see if that aids in identification. Finally, the taster can unpinch the nose to see if that helps to identify the food. Some food suggestions include small pieces of fruit or vegetables, onion, nuts, or chocolate.

Important notes:

a. Make sure you check for any students with food allergies before beginning this activity.

b. Make sure you are working in a clean environment.

c. Students might want to wear sterile gloves when handling the food items.

II. Are We Really What We Eat? (p. 87)

a. Atoms Bond to Form Molecules

b. Food Is Composed of Molecules

c. Molecules Join to Form Cells

d. Cells Join to Form Tissues and Organs

e. Organs Make Up Functional Systems

Key Terms: cell, cell membrane, cytoplasm, organelle, tissue, organ, system

Instructor Tools: Chapter 3 PPT slides, TAs 50–51

Images:

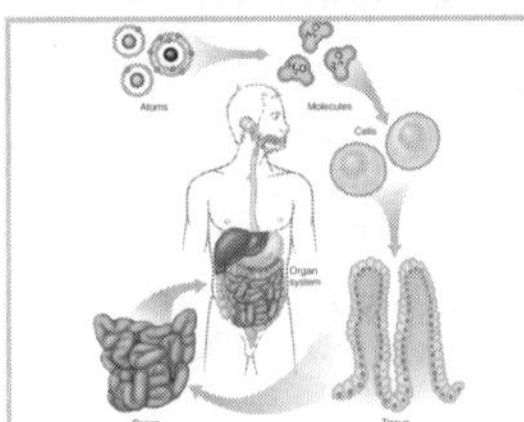

Figure 3.3
The organization of the human body.

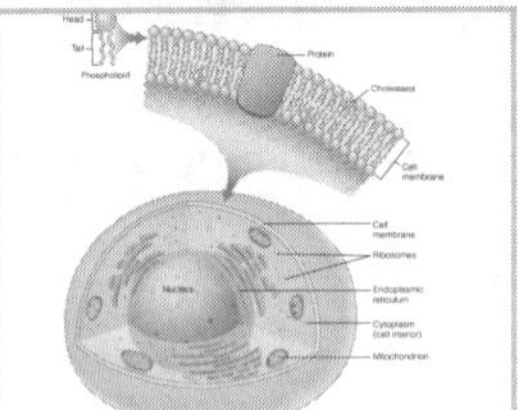

Figure 3.4
Representative cell of the small intestine.

III. What Happens to the Food We Eat? (p. 90)

a. Digestion Begins in the Mouth

b. The Esophagus Propels Food Into the Stomach

c. The Stomach Mixes, Digests, and Stores Food

d. Most Digestion and Absorption Occurs in the Small Intestine

e. The Large Intestine Stores Food Waste Until It Is Excreted

Key Terms: digestion, absorption, elimination, gastrointestinal (GI) tract, sphincter, cephalic phase, saliva, salivary glands, enzymes, bolus, esophagus, peristalsis, stomach, gastric juice, denature, chyme, small intestine, gallbladder, pancreas, lacteal, brush border, liver, large intestine

Instructor Tools: Chapter 3 PPT slides, Chapter 3 PRS Clicker Questions slides 2–4, TAs 52–60

Animation: *Overview of Digestion & Absorption*

Images:

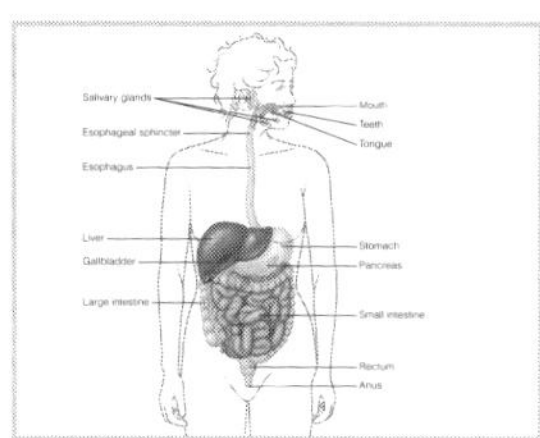

Figure 3.5
An overview of the gastrointestinal (GI) tract.

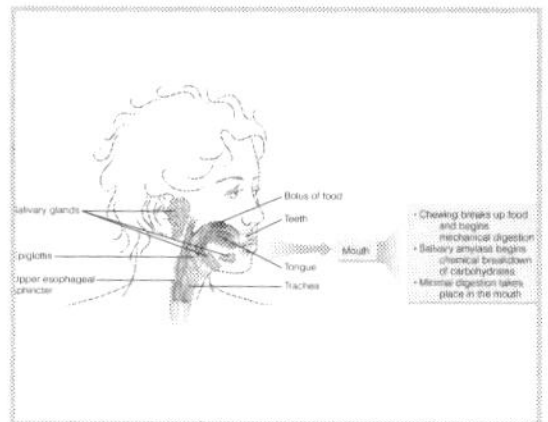

Figure 3.6
Where your food is now: the mouth.

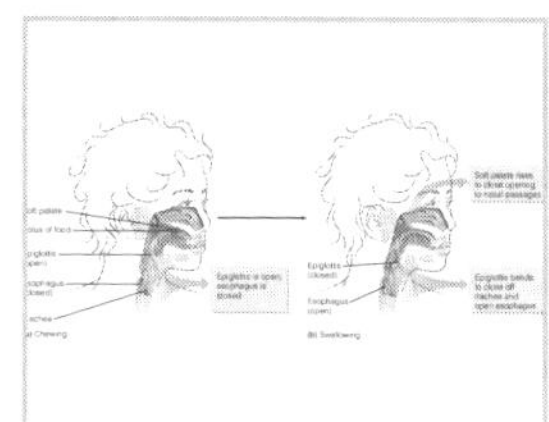

Figure 3.7
Chewing and swallowing are complex processes.

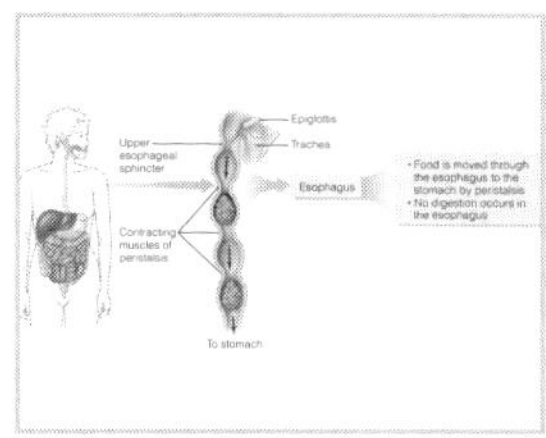

Figure 3.8
Where your food is now: the esophagus.

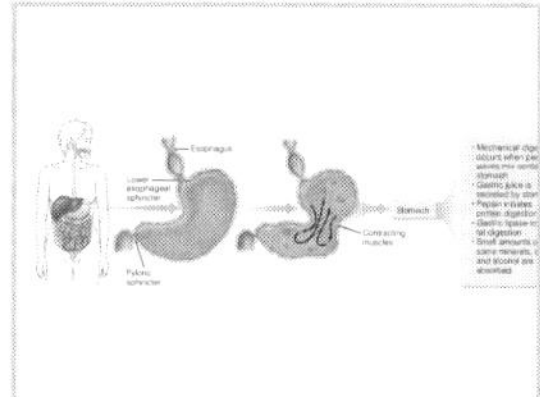

Figure 3.9
Where your food is now: the stomach.

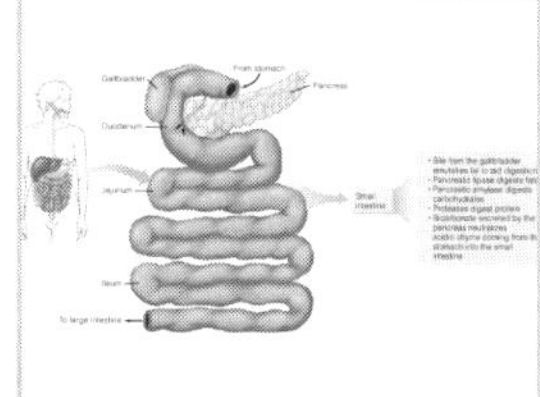

Figure 3.10
Where your food is now: the small intestine.

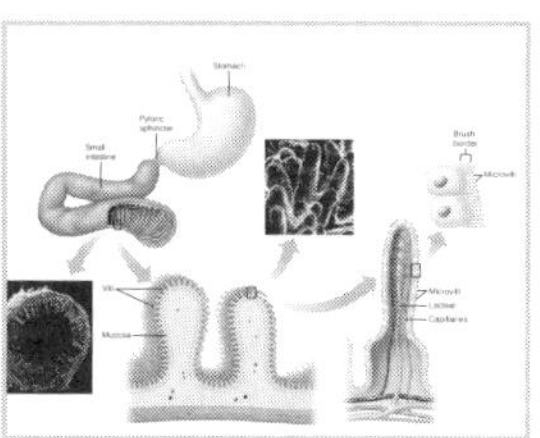

Figure 3.11
Absorption of nutrients occurs via the specialized lining of the small intestine.

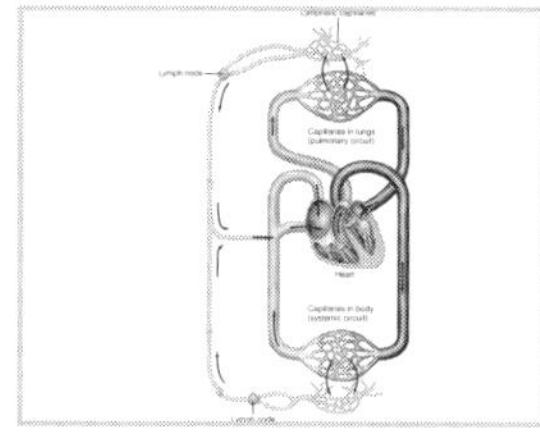

Figure 3.12
The cardiovascular and lymphatic systems.

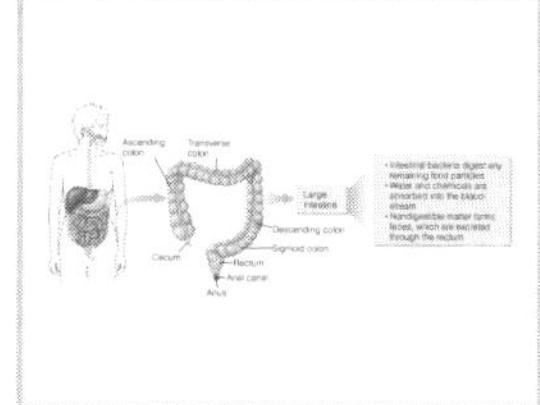

Figure 3.13
Where your food is now: the large intestine.

Activities:

1. Spread a continuous length of paper (such as butcher paper) approximately 15 feet long on the floor. Have students mark off appropriate lengths for each organ in the GI tract. Have students summarize the digestive activities that occur in each organ.
2. Demonstrate the Heimlich maneuver. Discuss when it is appropriate to perform this maneuver and the dangers of being too forceful.

IV. How Does the Body Coordinate and Regulate Digestion? (p. 101)

a. The Muscles of the Gastrointestinal Tract Mix and Move Food

b. The Enteric Nerves Coordinate and Regulate Digestive Activities

Key Term: enteric nervous system

Instructor Tools: Chapter 3 PPT slides

V. What Disorders Are Related to Digestion, Absorption, and Elimination?

a. Heartburn Is Caused by Reflux of Stomach Acid

b. An Ulcer Is an Area of Erosion in the GI Tract

c. Some People Experience Disorders Related to Specific Foods

d. Diarrhea and Constipation

e. Irritable Bowel Syndrome

Key Terms: heartburn, gastroesophageal reflux disease (GERD), peptic ulcer, food intolerance, food allergy, celiac disease, diarrhea, constipation, irritable bowel syndrome

Instructor Tools: Chapter 3 PPT slides, Chapter 3 PRS Clicker Questions slide 5, TAs 61–64

Images:

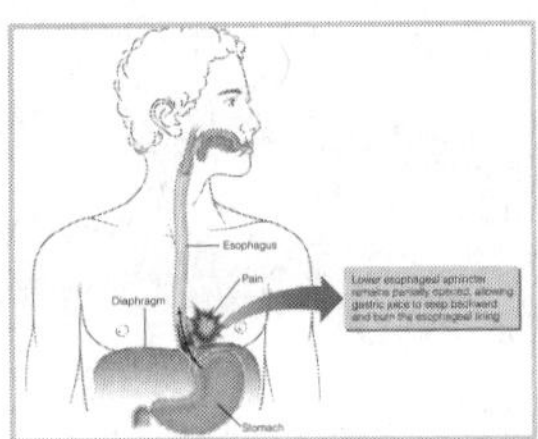

Figure 3.14
The mechanism of heartburn and gastroesophageal reflux disease.

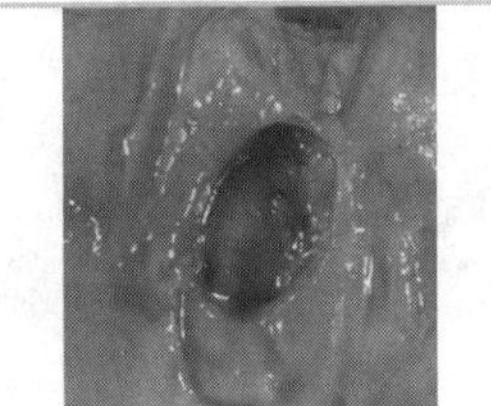

Figure 3.15
A peptic ulcer.

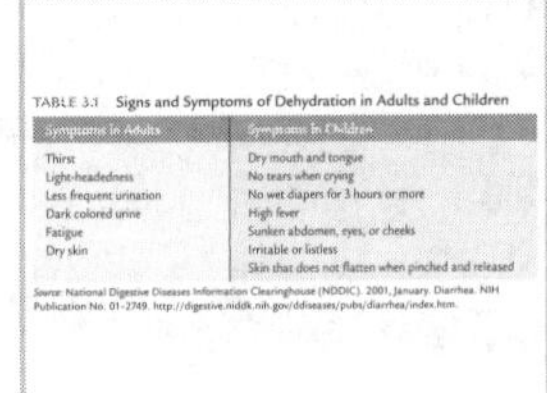

TABLE 3.1 Signs and Symptoms of Dehydration in Adults and Children

Symptoms in Adults	Symptoms in Children
Thirst	Dry mouth and tongue
Light-headedness	No tears when crying
Less frequent urination	No wet diapers for 3 hours or more
Dark colored urine	High fever
Fatigue	Sunken abdomen, eyes, or cheeks
Dry skin	Irritable or listless
	Skin that does not flatten when pinched and released

Source: National Digestive Diseases Information Clearinghouse (NDDIC). 2001, January. Diarrhea. NIH Publication No. 01-2749. http://digestive.niddk.nih.gov/ddiseases/pubs/diarrhea/index.htm.

Table 3.1
Signs and Symptoms of Dehydration in Adults and Children

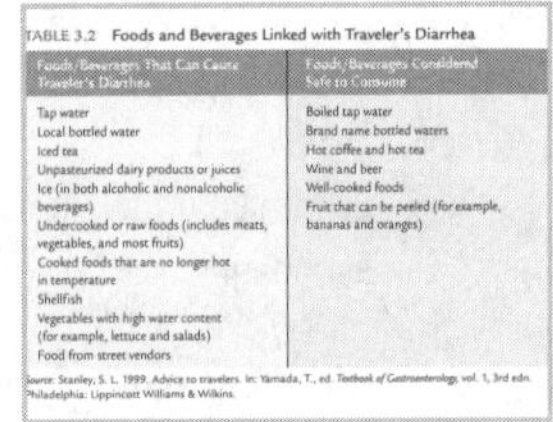

TABLE 3.2 Foods and Beverages Linked with Traveler's Diarrhea

Foods/Beverages That Can Cause Traveler's Diarrhea	Foods/Beverages Considered Safe to Consume
Tap water	Boiled tap water
Local bottled water	Brand name bottled waters
Iced tea	Hot coffee and hot tea
Unpasteurized dairy products or juices	Wine and beer
Ice (in both alcoholic and nonalcoholic beverages)	Well-cooked foods
Undercooked or raw foods (includes meats, vegetables, and most fruits)	Fruit that can be peeled (for example, bananas and oranges)
Cooked foods that are no longer hot in temperature	
Shellfish	
Vegetables with high water content (for example, lettuce and salads)	
Food from street vendors	

Source: Stanley, S. L. 1999. Advice to travelers. In: Yamada, T., ed. *Textbook of Gastroenterology,* vol. 1, 3rd edn. Philadelphia: Lippincott Williams & Wilkins.

Table 3.2
Foods and Beverages Linked to Traveler's Diarrhea

Activity:

Have students bring to class or research on the Internet over-the-counter products used to treat digestive difficulties such as heartburn, diarrhea, and constipation. Discuss the advantages and disadvantages of taking these products. Ask students if they can come up with any alternative ideas for addressing these problems.

VI. Additional Chapter 3 Instructor Tools

MyDietAnalysis Activity: The health of the GI tract depends to a great extent on the foods we eat. Using the nutritional assessment previously completed, students should review the information provided by their diet analysis software and note the following:

1. Do you meet recommendations for fiber intake?
2. Do you meet recommendations for water intake?
3. If you have any GI difficulties, can you correlate them with any of the foods you consume?
4. What changes could you make in your diet to improve the health of your GI tract?

Nutrition Debate Activity: Have students plan a gluten free menu. You may want to assign different meals to different students to get a variety of ideas. Explain that gluten can hide in many processed foods and that ingredients must be carefully checked to ensure that they are free of all gluten.

Printed TestBank: Pages 28–41 (TestGen Chapter 3)

Quiz Show PowerPoints: Chapter 3

Notes

Carbohydrates: Plant-Derived Energy Nutrients 4

Chapter at a Glance

I. What Are Carbohydrates?
II. What's the Difference Between Simple and Complex Carbohydrates?
III. Why Do We Need Carbohydrates?
IV. How Do Our Bodies Break Down Carbohydrates?
V. How Much Carbohydrate Should We Eat?
VI. What's the Story on Alternative Sweeteners?
VII. What Disorders Are Related to Carbohydrate Metabolism?

Visual Lecture Outline

I. What Are Carbohydrates? (p. 118)

Key Terms: carbohydrate, glucose, photosynthesis

Instructor Tools: Chapter 4 PPT slides, TA 65

Image:

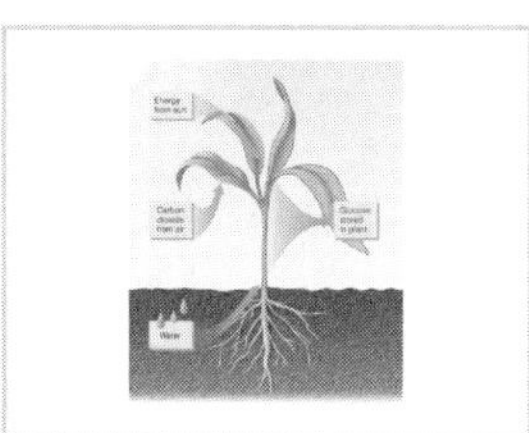

Figure 4.1
Plants make carbohydrates through the process of photosynthesis.

II. What's the Difference Between Simple and Complex Carbohydrates? (p. 118)

a. Simple Carbohydrates Include Monosaccharides and Disaccharides
b. All Complex Carbohydrates Are Polysaccharides

Key Terms: simple carbohydrate, monosaccharide, disaccharide, fructose, galactose, lactose, maltose, sucrose, complex carbohydrate, polysaccharide, starch, glycogen, dietary fiber, functional fiber, total fiber, soluble fiber, viscous, insoluble fibers

Instructor Tools: Chapter 4 PPT slides, Chapter 4 PRS Clicker Questions slides 1–2, TAs 66–68, 89

Images:

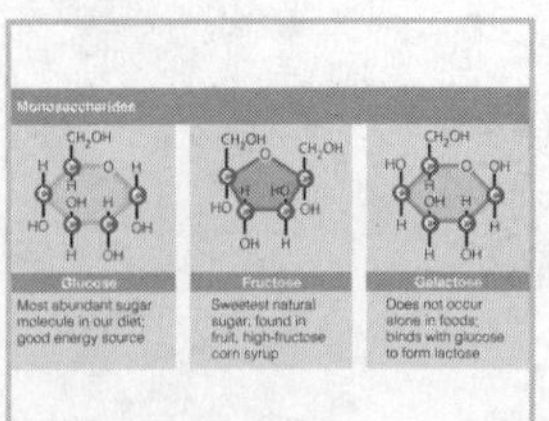

Figure 4.2
The three most common monosaccharides.

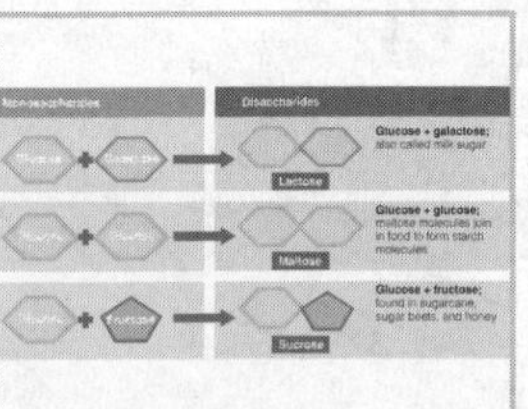

Figure 4.3
Galactose, glucose, and fructose join together to make the disaccharides lactose, maltose, and sucrose.

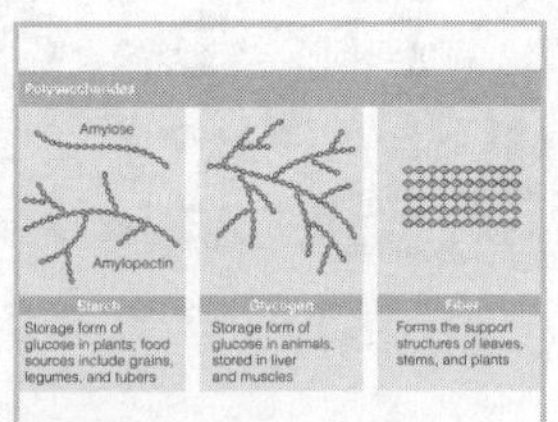

Figure 4.4
Polysaccharides include starch, glycogen, and fiber.

TABLE 4.1 Nutrient Comparison of Four Different Sugars

	Table Sugar	Raw Sugar	Honey	Molasses
Energy (kcal)	49	48.8	64	58
Carbohydrate (g)	12.60	12.6	17.3	14.95
Fat (g)	0	0	0	0.02
Protein (g)	0	0	0.06	0
Fiber (grams)	0	0	0	0
Vitamin C (mg)	0	0	0.1	0
Vitamin A (IU)	0	0	0	0
Thiamin (mg)	0	0	0	0.008
Riboflavin (mg)	0.002	0.003	0.008	0
Folate (µg)	0	0	0	0
Calcium (mg)	0	0.042	1	41
Iron (mg)	0	0	0.09	0.94
Sodium (mg)	0	0	1	7
Potassium (mg)	0	0.25	11	293

Source: U.S. Department of Agriculture, Agricultural Research Service. 2006. USDA National Nutrient Database for Standard Reference, Release 19. Nutrient Data Laboratory Home Page, http://www.ars.usda.gov/ba/bhnrc/ndl.
Note: Nutrient values are identified for one tablespoon of each product.

Table 4.1
Nutrient Comparison of Four Different Sugar

III. Why Do We Need Carbohydrates? (p. 124)

a. Carbohydrates Provide Energy
b. Complex Carbohydrates Have Health Benefits
c. Fiber Helps Us Stay Healthy

Key Terms: ketosis, ketones, ketoacidosis, gluconeogenesis

Instructor Tools: Chapter 4 PPT slides, TAs 69–71

Animation: *Diverticulosis and Fiber*

Images:

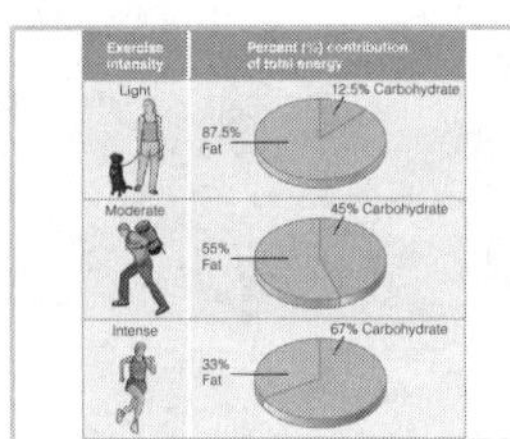

Figure 4.5
Amounts of carbohydrate and fat used during light, moderate, and intense exercise.

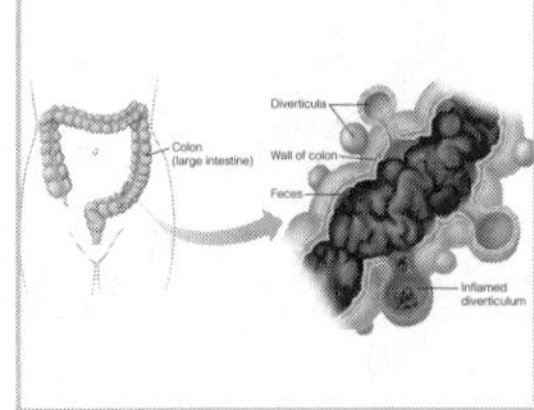

Figure 4.6
Diverticulosis occurs when bulging pockets form in the wall of the colon.

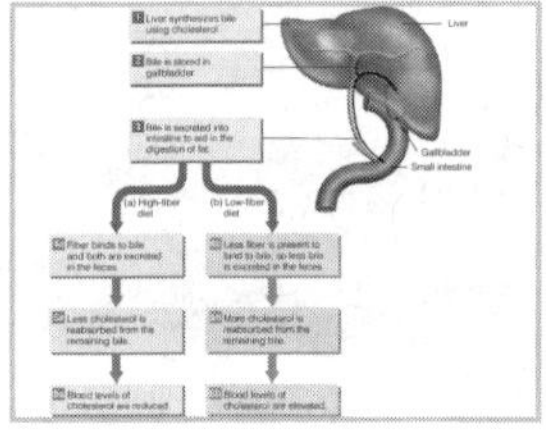

Figure 4.7
How fiber might help decrease blood cholesterol levels.

IV. How Do Our Bodies Break Down Carbohydrates? (p. 128)

a. Digestion Breaks Down Most Carbohydrates into Monosaccharides
b. The Liver Converts All Monosaccharides into Glucose
c. Fiber Is Excreted from the Large Intestine
d. Insulin and Glucagon Regulate the Level of Glucose in Our Blood
e. The Glycemic Index Shows How Foods Affect Our Blood Glucose Levels

Key Terms: salivary amylase, pancreatic amylase, maltase, sucrase, lactase, insulin, glucagon, glycemic index, glycemic load

Instructor Tools: Chapter 4 PPT slides, Chapter 4 PRS Clicker Questions slides 3–4, TAs 72–76

Animations: *Carbohydrate Digestion, Carbohydrate Absorption, Hormonal Control of Blood Glucose*

Images:

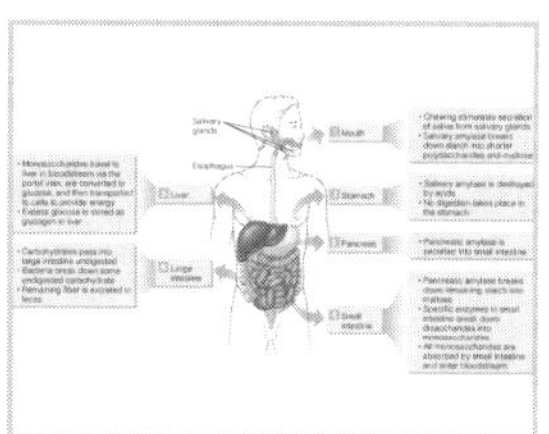

Figure 4.8
A review of carbohydrate digestion and absorption.

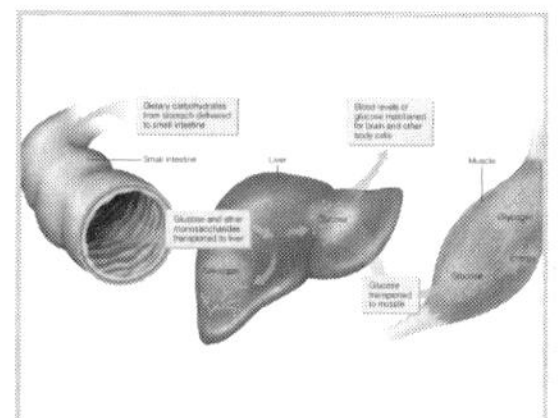

Figure 4.9
Glucose is stored as glycogen in both liver and muscle.

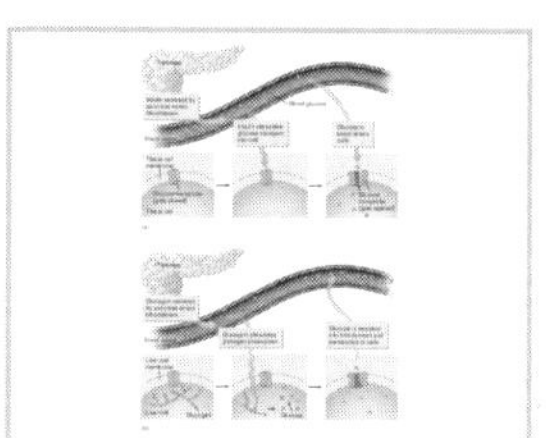

Figure 4.10
Regulation of blood glucose by the hormones insulin and glucagon.

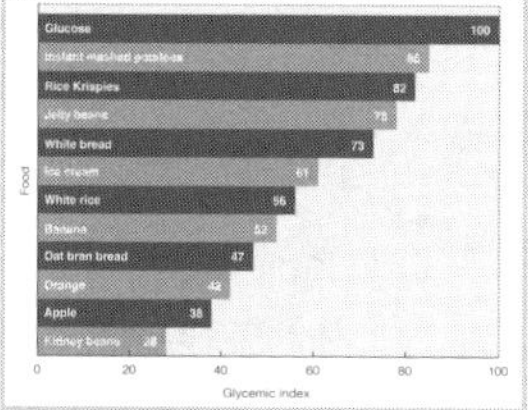

Figure 4.11
Glycemic index values for various foods as compared to pure glucose.

V. How Much Carbohydrate Should We Eat? (p. 134)

a. Most Americans Eat Too Much Simple Carbohydrate
b. Most Americans Eat Too Little Complex Carbohydrate
c. Shopper's Guide: Hunting for Complex Carbohydrates

abc NEWS **Lecture Launcher Video:**

Whole Grains

abc NEWS **Video Discussion Questions:**

1. What is a "whole grain"?
2. What are some methods food manufacturers use to convince consumers that their products contain significant amounts of whole grain?
3. Are all products labeled as "whole grain" healthy? Explain.

abc NEWS **Lecture Launcher Video:**

Sugar and Processed Foods

abc NEWS **Video Discussion Questions:**

1. What are some of the concerns regarding processed foods?
2. How has the food industry responded to the concerns about their products?
3. Are low fat products the best choice for weight loss? Why or why not?

Key Term: added sugars

Instructor Tools: Chapter 4 PPT slides, Chapter 4 PRS Clicker Questions slide 5, TAs 77–84, 90–91

Images:

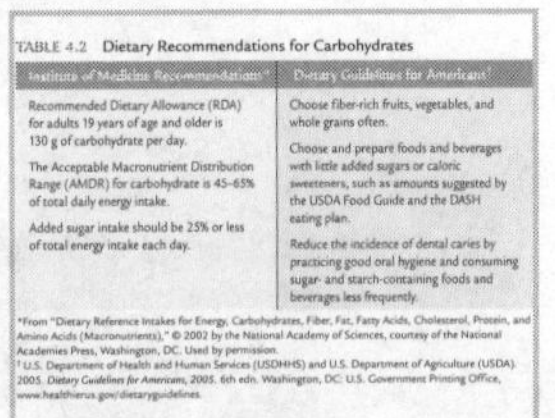

Table 4.2
Dietary Recommendations for Carbohydrates

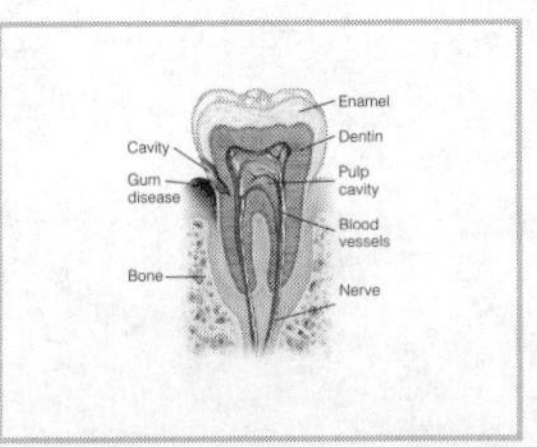

Figure 4.12
Eating simple carbohydrates can cause an increase in cavities and gum disease.

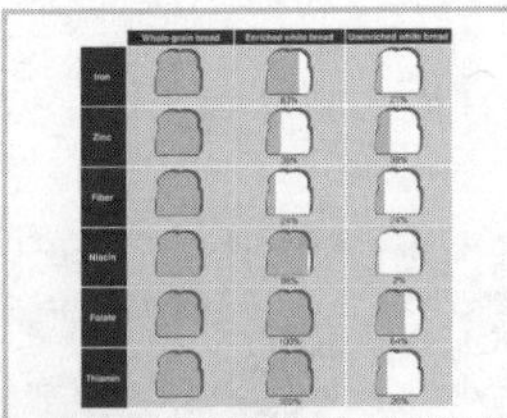

Figure 4.13
Nutrients in whole-grain, enriched white, and unenriched white breads.

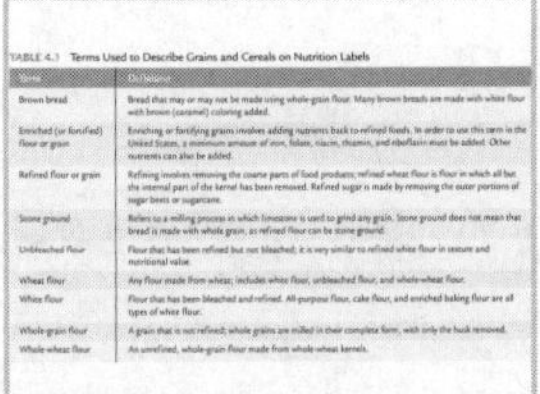

Table 4.3
Terms Used to Describe Grains and Cereals on Nutrition Labels

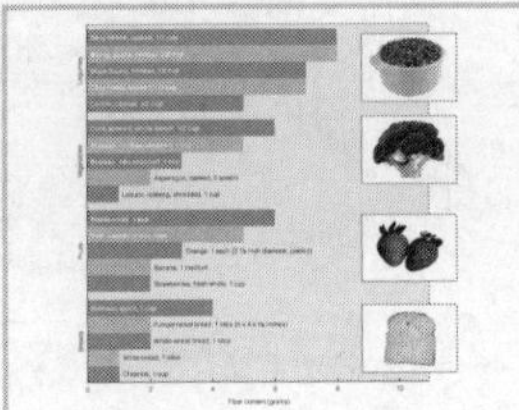

Figure 4.14
Fiber content of common foods.

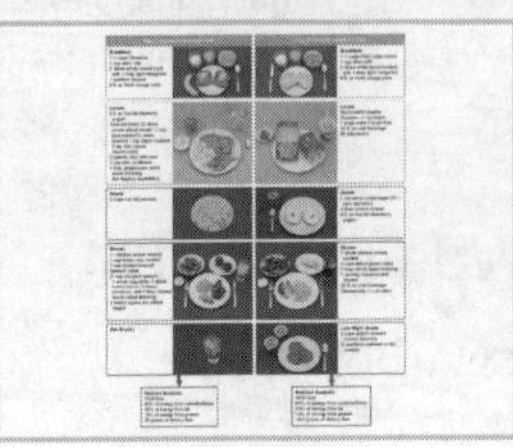

Figure 4.15
Comparison of two high-carbohydrate diets.

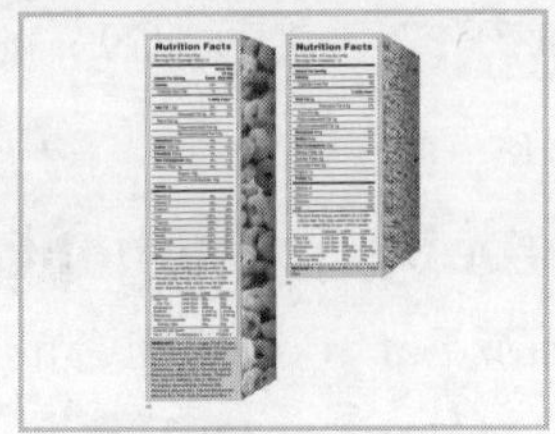

Figure 4.16
Labels for two breakfast cereals. (a) Sweetened cereal. (b) Whole-grain cereal.

Activities:

1. Have students bring to class the Nutrition Facts label of their favorite cereal. Make a list on the board containing the following information for each cereal:
   a. the number of calories per serving
   b. the amount of sugar per serving
   c. the amount of fiber per serving

   Discuss which cereals represent the best choices. You may want to review the concept of nutrient density during this discussion. Instruct students to examine the ingredients list to see where sugar falls. Remind them that the ingredients are listed in descending order by weight. Review all the terms that denote sugar and explain to students that many manufacturers list the different forms of sugar separately so they will appear further down the list. However, if all forms of sugar are added up, this may still be the ingredient present in the highest amount.
2. Ask students to bring 2 to 3 of their favorite foods to class. You will need to make sugar, scales, and/or measuring tools available to them. Have them work in groups, weighing or measuring the amount of sugar in each food. This helps students visualize the quantities of sugar in foods.

VI. What's the Story on Alternative Sweeteners? (p. 143)

a. Alternative Sweeteners Are Non-Nutritive
b. Limited Use of Alternative Sweeteners Is Not Harmful

Key Terms: nutritive sweeteners, non-nutritive sweeteners, acceptable daily intake (ADI)

Instructor Tools: Chapter 4 PPT slides, TAs 85, 92

Images:

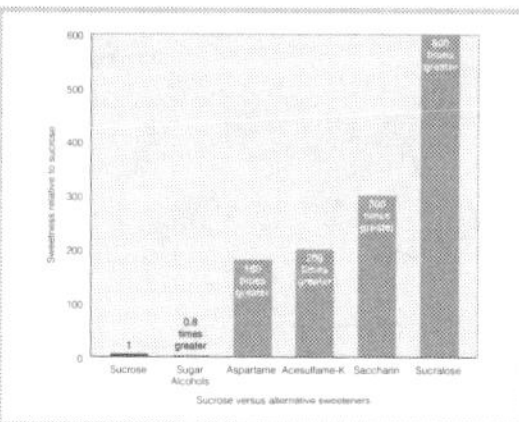

Figure 4.17
Relative sweetness of alternative sweeteners as compared to sucrose.

TABLE 4.4 The Amount of Food that a 50-Pound Child and a 150-Pound Adult Would Have to Consume Each Day to Exceed the ADI for Aspartame

Food	50-Pound Child	150-Pound Adult
12 fl. oz carbonated soft drink	7	20
8 fl. oz powdered soft drink	11	34
4 fl. oz gelatin dessert	14	42
Packets of tabletop sweetener	32	97

Source: Adapted from International Food Information Council. 2001. *Food Safety and Nutrition Information Sweeteners. Everything You Need to Know about Aspartame.* http://ific.org/publications/factsheets/lcsfs.cfm

Table 4.4
The Amount of Food that a 50-Pound Child and a 150-Pound Adult Would Have to Consume Each Day to Exceed the ADI For Aspartame

VII. What Disorders Are Related to Carbohydrate Metabolism? (p. 146)

a. Diabetes: Impaired Regulation of Glucose
b. Hypoglycemia: Low Blood Glucose
c. Lactose Intolerance: Inability to Digest Lactose

Key Terms: diabetes, type 1 diabetes, type 2 diabetes, impaired fasting glucose, hypoglycemia, lactose intolerance

Instructor Tools: Chapter 4 PPT slides, Chapter 4 PRS Clicker Questions slide 6, TAs 86–88, 93

Images:

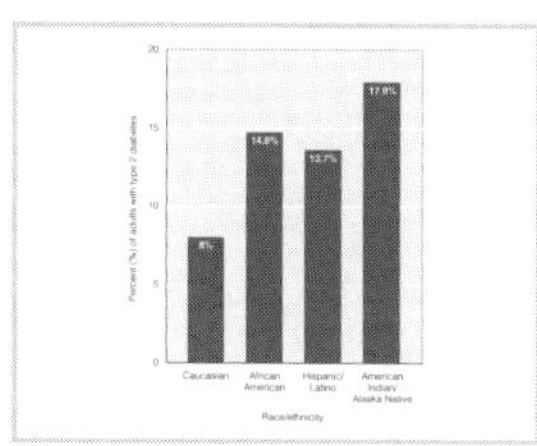

Figure 4.18
The percent of adults from various ethnic and racial groups with type 2 diabetes.

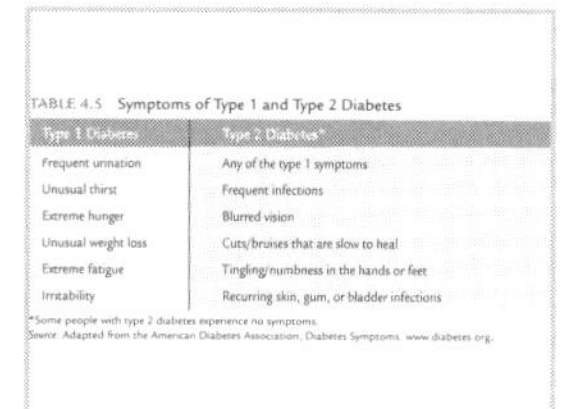

TABLE 4.5 Symptoms of Type 1 and Type 2 Diabetes

Type 1 Diabetes	Type 2 Diabetes*
Frequent urination	Any of the type 1 symptoms
Unusual thirst	Frequent infections
Extreme hunger	Blurred vision
Unusual weight loss	Cuts/bruises that are slow to heal
Extreme fatigue	Tingling/numbness in the hands or feet
Irritability	Recurring skin, gum, or bladder infections

*Some people with type 2 diabetes experience no symptoms.
Source: Adapted from the American Diabetes Association, Diabetes Symptoms. www.diabetes.org.

Table 4.5
Symptoms of Type 1 and Type 2 Diabetes

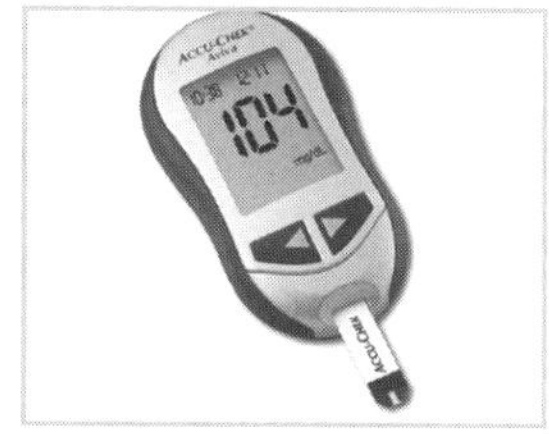

Figure 4.19
Monitoring blood glucose requires pricking the fingers each day and measuring the blood using a glucometer.

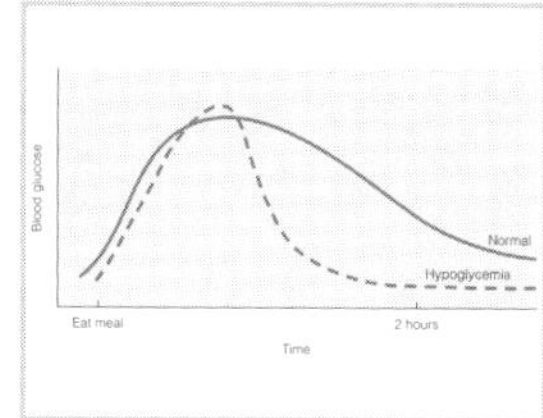

Figure 4.20
Changes in blood glucose after a meal for people with hypoglycemia and without hypoglycemia (normal).

Activities:

1. Have each student bring in an article on diabetes from a newspaper, magazine, or the Internet. Students should summarize the information in their article for the class. This activity can lead to further discussion about diabetes, if desired.
2. Have students plan a one-day menu for an individual with lactose intolerance.

VIII. Additional Chapter 4 Instructor Tools

MyDietAnalysis Activity: Using the nutritional assessment previously completed, students should note the following:

1. How many grams of carbohydrate do you consume daily?
2. What percentage of your daily calories come from carbohydrate?
3. How many grams of sugar do you consume daily?
4. What percentage of your daily calories come from sugar?
5. Do your intakes meet recommendations for these nutrients?
6. What three foods did you consume that contain the highest level of sugar? How many grams of sugar were in each food?
7. What changes can you make in your diet to more closely meet carbohydrate and sugar recommendations?

Nutrition Debate Activity: For this demonstration, you will need a teaspoon, sugar, and a clear glass. Ask students how much sugar they put in coffee or tea. Start adding sugar to the glass as students offer their suggestions. When you reach the maximum amount of sugar suggested by students, note the amount you added. Continue adding sugar until you have added 10 teaspoons. Hold the glass up and ask if students would drink a liquid poured into the glass with that much sugar. Explain that it is the amount of sugar in a can of soda.

Printed TestBank: Pages 42–55 (TestGen Chapter 4)

Quiz Show PowerPoints: Chapter 4

In Depth: Alcohol

Chapter at a Glance

I. What Are the Health Benefits and Concerns of Moderate Alcohol Intake?
II. How Is Alcohol Metabolized?
III. Effects of Excessive Alcohol Intake on Personal Health
IV. Should You Be Concerned About Your Alcohol Intake?
V. Talking to Someone About Alcohol Addiction

Visual Lecture Outline

I. What Are the Health Benefits and Concerns of Moderate Alcohol Intake? (p. 116)

a. Benefits of Moderate Alcohol Intake

b. Concerns of Moderate Alcohol Intake

Key Terms: alcohol, ethanol, drink, proof, resveratrol

Instructor Tools: In Depth: Alcohol PPT slides, In Depth: Alcohol PRS Clicker Questions slides 1–2, TA 94

Image:

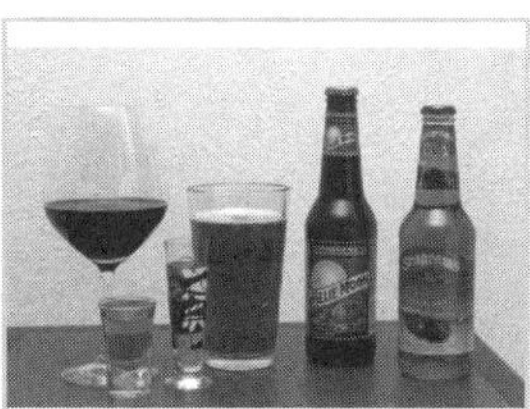

Figure 1
What does one drink look like?

Activity:

Perform the following demonstration to illustrate that the amount of alcohol in 12 ounces of beer is the same as in 5 ounces of wine and the same as in 1½ ounces of hard liquor:

Bring to class a shot glass, a wine glass, and a beer mug.

Fill four 1-gallon containers about ¾ full of water. Add about 1 teaspoon of red food coloring to one of the gallon containers and mix. The food coloring represents the alcohol.

Add 1½ ounces of the diluted food coloring mixture to the shot glass.

Add 1½ ounces of the diluted food coloring mixture to the wine glass which also contains 3½ ounces of water (5 ounces total).

Add 1½ ounces of the diluted food coloring mixture to the beer mug which also contains 10 ½ ounces of water (12 ounces total).

Ask students to discuss how the amount of alcohol in each "drink" compares to the others and if the effects of each "drink" would differ from another.

To further illustrate that the effects of all 3 "drinks" would be the same, pour the contents of each one into a different gallon container of water. Explain the containers of water represent the bloodstream. Have students observe the color of all 3 containers with their "drinks" added. Since the color intensity of all containers will be the same (despite a slight difference in volume), it should be evident that the amount of food coloring (alcohol) in each container is the same.

II. How Is Alcohol Metabolized? (p. 162)

Instructor Tools: In Depth: Alcohol PPT slides, In Depth: Alcohol PRS Clicker Questions slides 3–4, TAs 95, 98

Animation: *Alcohol Absorption*

Images:

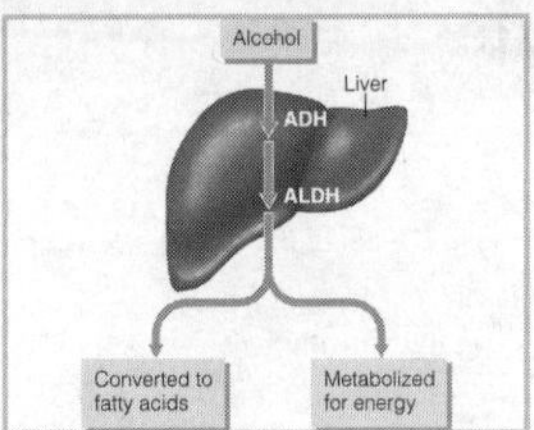

Figure 2
Metabolism of alcohol.

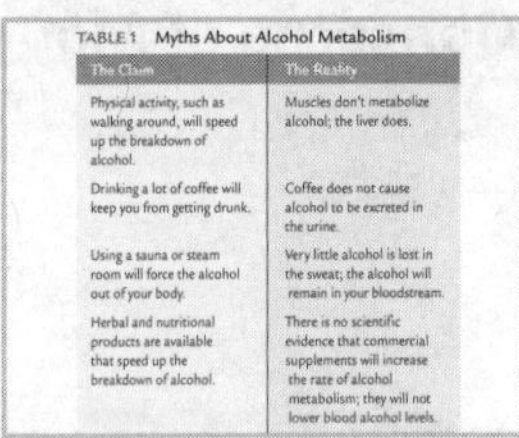

TABLE 1 Myths About Alcohol Metabolism

The Claim	The Reality
Physical activity, such as walking around, will speed up the breakdown of alcohol.	Muscles don't metabolize alcohol; the liver does.
Drinking a lot of coffee will keep you from getting drunk.	Coffee does not cause alcohol to be excreted in the urine.
Using a sauna or steam room will force the alcohol out of your body.	Very little alcohol is lost in the sweat; the alcohol will remain in your bloodstream.
Herbal and nutritional products are available that speed up the breakdown of alcohol.	There is no scientific evidence that commercial supplements will increase the rate of alcohol metabolism; they will not lower blood alcohol levels.

Table 1
Myths About Alcohol Metabolism

III. Effects of Excessive Alcohol Intake on Personal Health (p. 164)

a. The Effects of Alcohol Hangovers
b. Reduced Brain Function
c. Reduced Liver Function
d. Increased Risk of Chronic Disease
e. Malnutrition
f. Increased Risk of Traumatic Injury
g. Fetal and Infant Health Problems

abc NEWS **Lecture Launcher Video:**

Women and Alcohol

abc NEWS **Video Discussion Questions:**

1. What are some factors that contribute to alcohol abuse in college-age women?
2. Discuss risks of alcohol abuse in college-age women.
3. What can be done to discourage alcohol abuse in college students?

Key Terms: binge drinking, alcohol poisoning, alcoholism, alcohol hangover, fatty liver, alcoholic hepatitis, cirrhosis of the liver, teratogen, fetal alcohol syndrome (FAS), fetal alcohol effects (FAE)

Instructor Tools: In Depth: Alcohol PPT slides, In Depth: Alcohol PRS Clicker Questions slide 5, TAs 96–97, 99

Images:

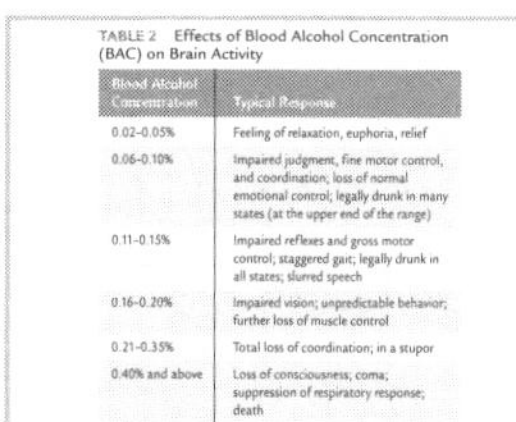

TABLE 2 Effects of Blood Alcohol Concentration (BAC) on Brain Activity

Blood Alcohol Concentration	Typical Response
0.02–0.05%	Feeling of relaxation, euphoria, relief
0.06–0.10%	Impaired judgment, fine motor control, and coordination; loss of normal emotional control; legally drunk in many states (at the upper end of the range)
0.11–0.15%	Impaired reflexes and gross motor control; staggered gait; legally drunk in all states; slurred speech
0.16–0.20%	Impaired vision; unpredictable behavior; further loss of muscle control
0.21–0.35%	Total loss of coordination; in a stupor
0.40% and above	Loss of consciousness; coma; suppression of respiratory response; death

Table 2
Effects of Blood Alcohol Concentration (BAC) on Brain Activity

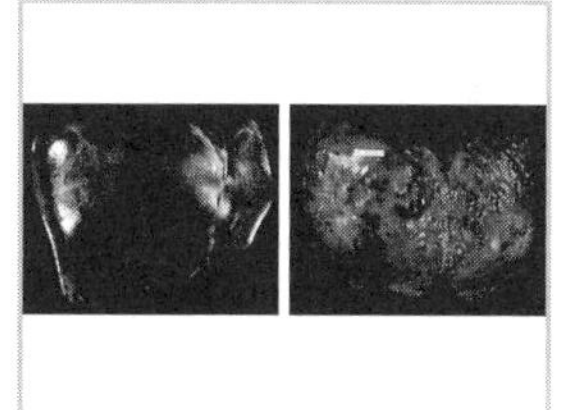

Figure 3
Cirrhosis of the liver, caused by chronic alcohol abuse.

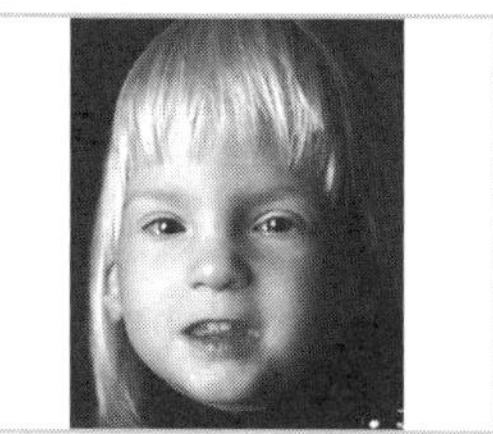

Figure 4
A child with fetal alcohol syndrome (FAS).

IV. Should You Be Concerned About Your Alcohol Intake? (p. 166)

Key Term: alcohol abuse

Instructor Tools: In Depth: Alcohol PPT slides

Activity:

Bring in alcohol advertisements from magazines. Divide the class into groups and have each group list ways that advertisers try to make alcohol seem desirable. Also have students note the age group that they feel is being targeted by the ad. Have one reporter from each group report their findings. Summarize the findings as a class and discuss how advertising influences the public.

V. Talking to Someone About Alcohol Addiction (p. 166)

Instructor Tools: In Depth: Alcohol PPT slides

VI. Additional In Depth: Alcohol Instructor Tools

MyDietAnalysis Activity: Using the nutritional assessment previously completed, students should note the following:

1. If you drank alcoholic beverages, how many drinks did you consume daily?
2. How many grams of alcohol did you average per day?
3. How many kilocalories came from alcohol? (Alcohol contains 7 kcalories per gram.)
4. What percentage of your energy intake comes from alcohol? Calculate using this formula:

   kcals from alcohol/total kcals × 100 = % kcals from alcohol

Printed TestBank: Pages 56–59 (TestGen In Depth: Alcohol)

Notes

Fats: Essential Energy-Supplying Nutrients 5

Chapter at a Glance

I. What Are Fats?
II. Why Do We Need Fats?
III. When Are Fats Harmful?
IV. How Do Our Bodies Process Fats?
V. How Much Fat Should We Eat?
VI. What Role Do Fats Play in Cardiovascular Disease and Cancer?

Visual Lecture Outline

I. What Are Fats? (p. 172)

a. Most of the Fats We Eat Are in the Form of Triglycerides
b. Different Forms of Triglycerides Can Damage or Preserve Our Health
c. Phospholipids Combine Lipids with Phosphate
d. Sterols Have a Ring Structure

Key Terms: lipids, triglyceride, fatty acids, glycerol, short-chain fatty acids, medium-chain fatty acids, long-chain fatty acids, saturated fatty acids (SFAs), monounsaturated fatty acids (MUFAs), polyunsaturated fatty acids (PUFAs), hydrogenation, essential fatty acids (EFAs), linoleic acid, alpha-linolenic acid, eicosapentaenoic acid (EPA), docosahexaenoic acid (DHA), phospholipids, sterols

Instructor Tools: Chapter 5 PPT slides, Chapter 5 PRS Clicker Questions slides 1–2, TAs 100–107, 118

Animations: *Fats in Food, Lipoproteins*

Images:

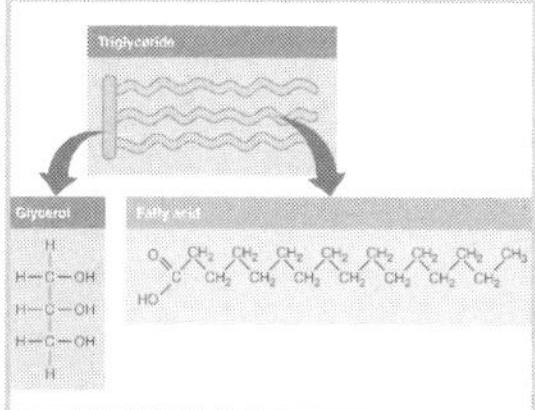

Figure 5.1
A triglyceride.

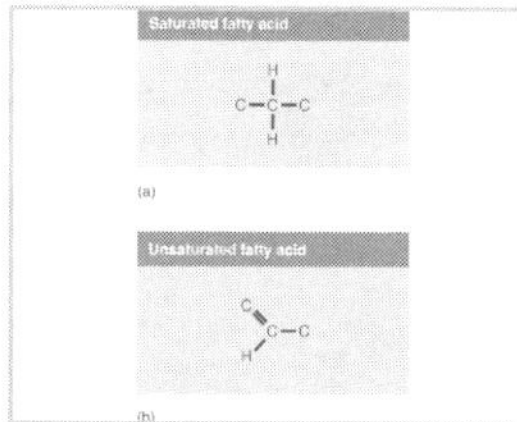

Figure 5.2
An atom of carbon has four attachment sites.

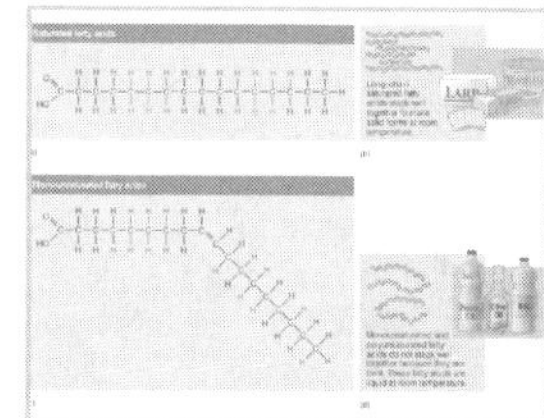
Figure 5.3
Level of saturation affects the shape of the fatty acids.

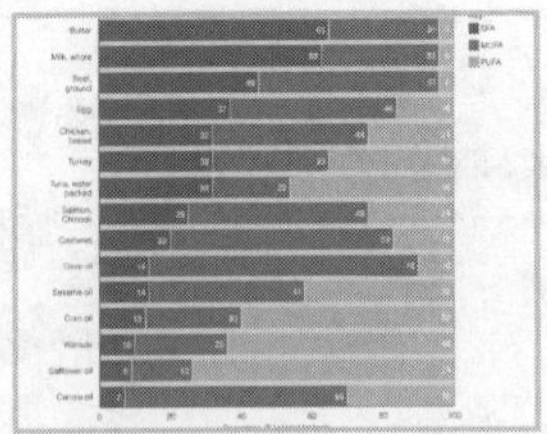

Figure 5.4
Major sources of dietary fat.

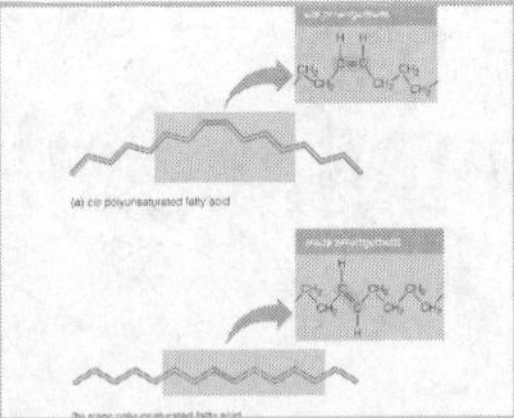

Figure 5.5
Structure of (a) a cis and (b) a *trans* polyunsaturated fatty acid.

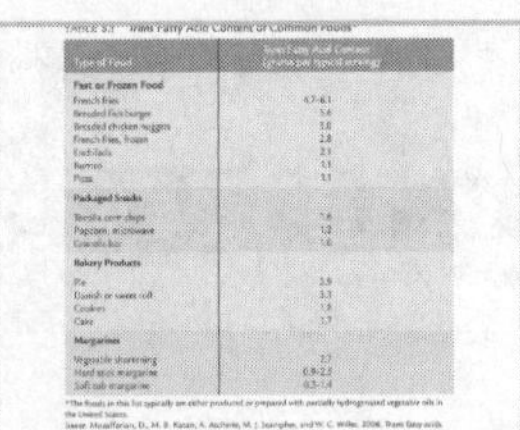

Table 5.1
Trans Fatty Acid Content of Common Foods

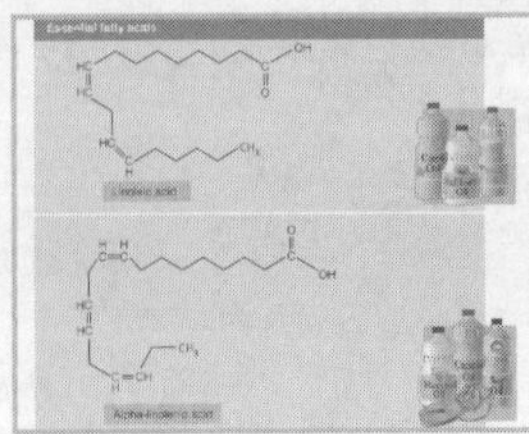

Figure 5.6
Linoleic acid (omega-6 fatty acid) and alpha-linolenic acid (omega-3 fatty acid).

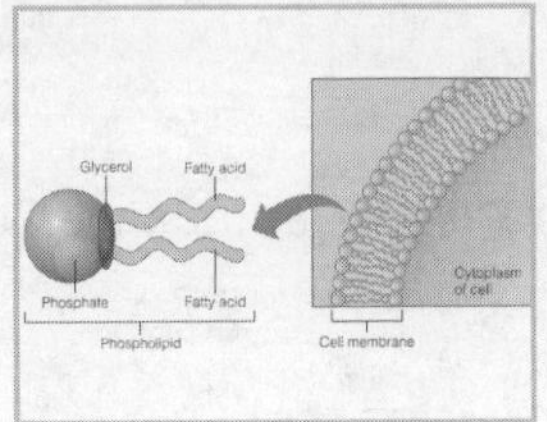

Figure 5.7
Structure of a phospholipid.

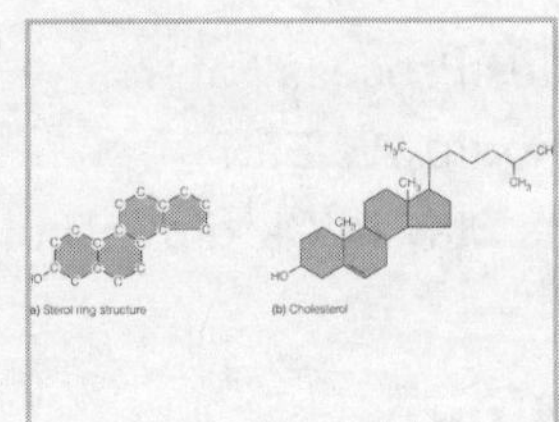

Figure 5.8
Sterol structure.

II. Why Do We Need Fats? (p. 181)

a. Fats Provide Energy
b. Body Fat Stores Energy for Later Use
c. Fats Enable the Transport of Fat-Soluble Vitamins
d. Fats Help Maintain Cell Function
e. Stored Fat Provides Protection to the Body
f. Fats Contribute to the Flavor and Texture of Foods
g. Fats Help Us to Feel Satiated

Instructor Tools: Chapter 5 PPT slides, TA 108

Image:

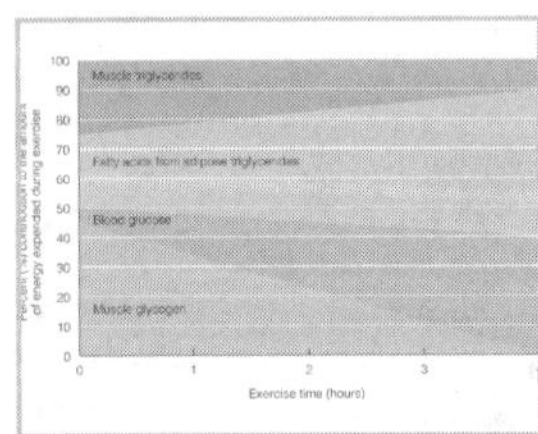

Figure 5.9
Various sources of energy used during exercise.

III. When Are Fats Harmful? (p. 184)

a. Eating Too Much of Certain Fats Can Lead to Disease

b. Fats Limit the Shelf Life of Foods

Instructor Tools: Chapter 5 PPT slides

IV. How Do Our Bodies Process Fats? (p. 185)

a. The Gallbladder, Liver, and Pancreas Assist in Fat Digestion

b. Absorption of Fat Occurs Primarily in the Small Intestine

c. Fat Is Stored in Adipose Tissues for Later Use

Key Terms: lipoprotein, chylomicron, lipoprotein lipase

Instructor Tools: Chapter 5 PPT slides, Chapter 5 PRS Clicker Questions slide 3, TAs 109–111

Animations: *Fat Digestion, Lipid Absorption*

Images:

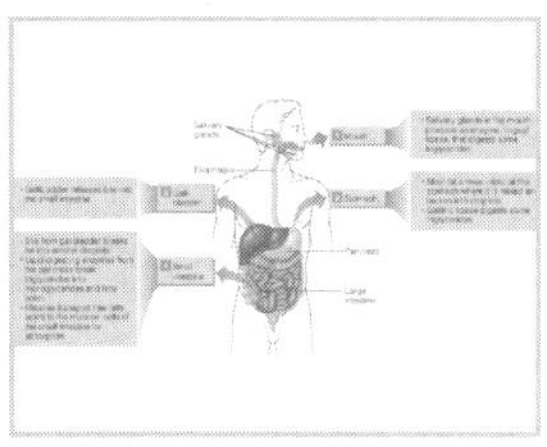

Figure 5.10
The process of fat digestion.

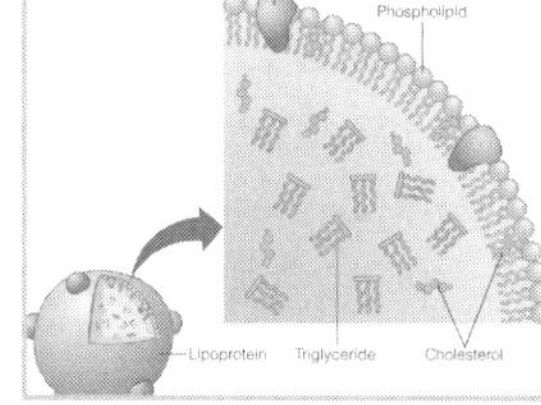

Figure 5.11
Structure of a lipoprotein.

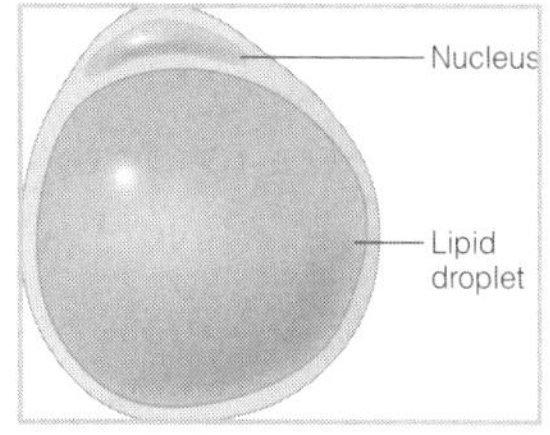

Figure 5.12
Diagram of an adipose cell.

Activity:

Mix oil and water together in a clear glass to demonstrate their immiscibility. Then add soap to the mixture to demonstrate the action of bile.

V. How Much Fat Should We Eat? (p. 187)

a. Dietary Reference Intake for Total Fat

b. Dietary Reference Intakes for Essential Fatty Acids

c. Most Americans Eat Within the Recommended Amount of Fat but Eat the Wrong Types

d. Food Sources of Fats

e. Shopper's Guide: Improving the Type and Quantity of Fat in Your Diet

abc NEWS **Lecture Launcher Video:**

Fast Food Trends

abc NEWS **Video Discussion Questions:**

1. What are some problems with "fast food" chicken?
2. Is it possible to get "healthy" fast food? Why or why not?
3. When you eat at a fast food restaurant, do you choose your meals based on health or taste? Do you think most other people use the same criteria as you do when choosing their meals?

Key Terms: visible fats, invisible fats

Instructor Tools: Chapter 5 PPT slides, Chapter 5 PRS Clicker Questions slide 4, TAs 113, 119–121

Images:

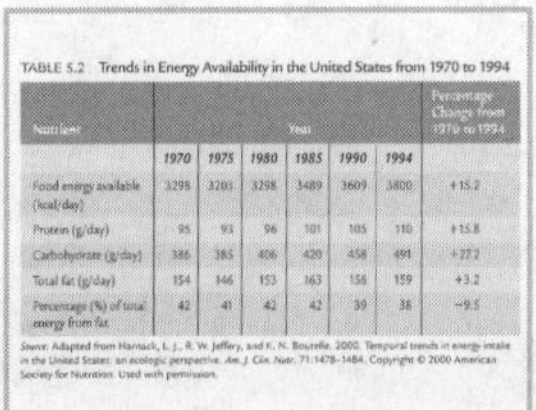

TABLE 5.2 Trends in Energy Availability in the United States from 1970 to 1994

Nutrient	Year						Percentage Change from 1970 to 1994
	1970	1975	1980	1985	1990	1994	
Food energy available (kcal/day)	3298	3203	3298	3489	3609	3800	+15.2
Protein (g/day)	95	93	96	101	105	110	+15.8
Carbohydrate (g/day)	386	385	406	420	458	491	+27.2
Total fat (g/day)	154	146	153	163	156	159	+3.2
Percentage (%) of total energy from fat	42	41	42	42	39	38	−9.5

Source: Adapted from Harnack, L. J., R. W. Jeffery, and K. N. Boutelle. 2000. Temporal trends in energy intake in the United States: an ecologic perspective. *Am. J. Clin. Nutr.* 71:1478–1484. Copyright © 2000 American Society for Nutrition. Used with permission.

Table 5.2
Trends in Energy Availability in the United States from 1970 to1994

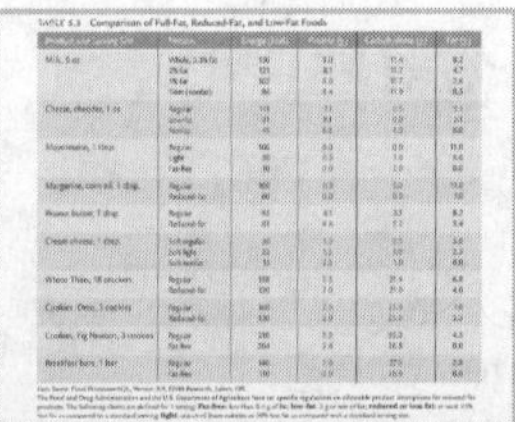

Table 5.3
Comparison of Full-Fat, Reduced-Fat, and Low-Fat Foods

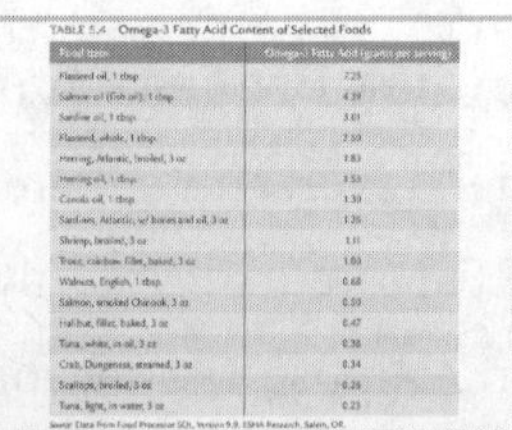

Table 5.4
Omega-3 Fatty Acid Content of Selected Foods

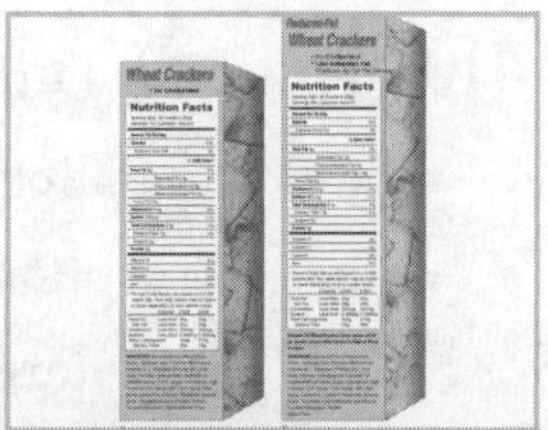

Figure 5.14
Labels for two types of wheat crackers. (a) Regular wheat crackers. (b) Reduced-fat wheat crackers.

Activities:

1. Instruct students to compare the amount of fat and calories in a baked, broiled, or steamed food compared to a fried food. The food composition table in the appendix can be used for this activity. Examples of foods to compare might be baked potatoes versus French fries, baked chicken versus fried chicken, broiled fish versus fried fish. Remind students to compare the same serving size of each food.
2. Ask each student to bring in a Nutrition Fact Sheet for his or her favorite order at a fast-food restaurant. Compile a list of the various foods, including:
   a. total calories
   b. calories from fat
   c. grams of fat
   d. grams of saturated fat
   e. percent of calories from fat (students will need to calculate this value: calories from fat ÷ total calories × 100)
3. Have students work in small groups to measure the amount of fat found in some of their favorite foods. Vegetable oil (1 Tbsp oil = 14 grams) can be measured into plastic cups for this activity. Students can use MyDietAnalysis software or Appendix A in their text to look up the amount of fat in the foods of interest.

VI. What Role Do Fats Play in Cardiovascular Disease and Cancer? (p. 195)

a. Fats Can Protect Against or Promote Cardiovascular Disease
b. Does a High-Fat Diet Cause Cancer?

Key Term: cardiovascular disease

Instructor Tools: Chapter 5 PPT slides, Chapter 5 PRS Clicker Questions slide 5, TAs 112, 114–117

Images:

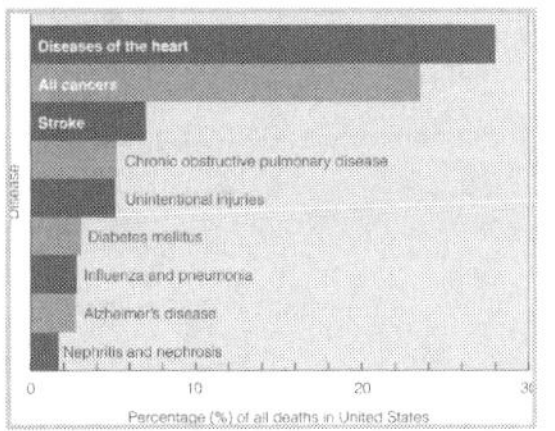

Figure 5.13
Cardiovascular disease, which includes heart disease, is the leading cause of death in the United States.

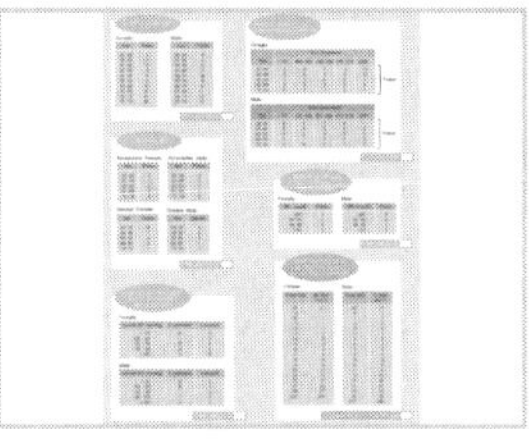

Figure 5.15
Calculation matrix to estimate the 10-year risk for cardiovascular disease for men and women.

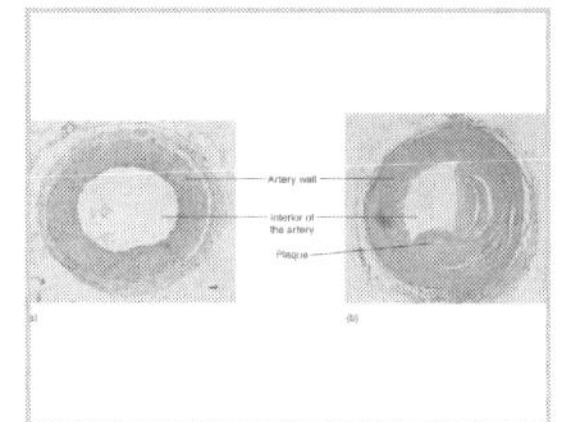

Figure 5.16
These light micrographs show a cross section of (a) a normal artery, and (b) an artery that is partially blocked with cholesterol-rich plaque.

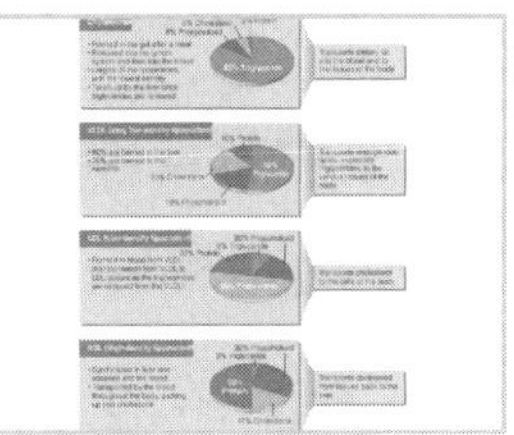

Figure 5.17
The chemical components of various lipoproteins.

Activity:

Have students work in small groups to develop a profile of an individual most likely to have a heart attack, including:

a. dietary habits

b. age

c. lifestyle

d. physical characteristics

Students should also offer suggestions on how to decrease the risk.

VII. Additional Chapter 5 Instructor Tools

MyDietAnalysis Activity: Using the nutritional assessment previously completed, students should note the following:

1. How many grams of fat do you consume daily?
2. What percentage of your daily calories come from fat?
3. How many grams of saturated fat do you consume daily?
4. How many grams of trans fat do you consume daily?
5. How many grams of cholesterol do you consume daily?
6. Do your intakes meet recommendations for these nutrients?
7. What three foods that you consumed contained the highest level of fat? How many grams of fat were in each food?
8. What changes can you make in your diet to more closely meet fat and cholesterol recommendations?

Nutrition Debate Activity: Instruct students to keep track of all the fast-food restaurants they pass on a normal day. Have them bring their lists to class and, working in small groups, discuss whether or not they believe eating at these restaurants can be a part of a healthful diet. Suggestions to include in this discussion are:

1. Is it ever appropriate to eat at these establishments? If so, who and when?
2. Are there food options available that can fit into a healthy diet? (To further research this question, students can actually visit the restaurant or investigate the restaurant website). Would you choose the healthy options?

3. If you were giving dietary advice, would you recommend these restaurants be totally avoided? Why or why not?

Printed TestBank: Pages 60–73 (TestGen Chapter 5)

Quiz Show PowerPoints: Chapter 5

Proteins: Crucial Components of All Body Tissues

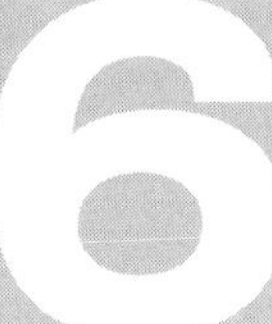

Chapter at a Glance

I. What Are Proteins?
II. How Are Proteins Made?
III. Why Do We Need Proteins?
IV. How Do Our Bodies Break Down Proteins?
V. How Much Proteins Should We Eat?
VI. Can a Vegetarian Diet Provide Adequate Protein?
VII. What Disorders Are Related to Protein Intake or Metabolism?

Visual Lecture Outline

I. What Are Proteins? (p. 212)

a. How Do Proteins Differ from Carbohydrates and Lipids?

b. The Building Blocks of Proteins Are Amino Acids

Key Terms: proteins, amino acids, essential amino acids, nonessential amino acids, transamination

Instructor Tools: Chapter 6 PPT slides, TAs 122–123, 138

Animation: *Protein Building Blocks*

Images:

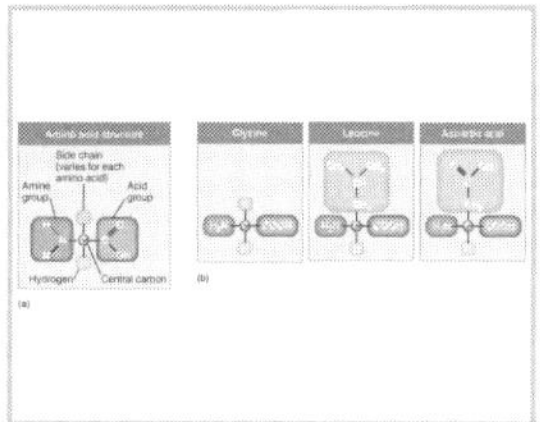

Figure 6.1
Structure of an amino acid.

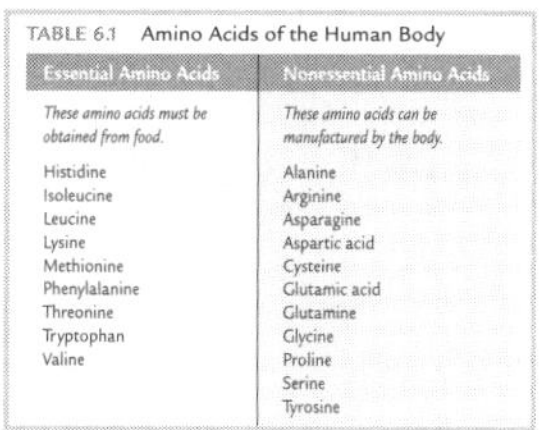

TABLE 6.1 Amino Acids of the Human Body

Essential Amino Acids	Nonessential Amino Acids
These amino acids must be obtained from food.	*These amino acids can be manufactured by the body.*
Histidine	Alanine
Isoleucine	Arginine
Leucine	Asparagine
Lysine	Aspartic acid
Methionine	Cysteine
Phenylalanine	Glutamic acid
Threonine	Glutamine
Tryptophan	Glycine
Valine	Proline
	Serine
	Tyrosine

Table 6.1
Amino Acids of the Human Body

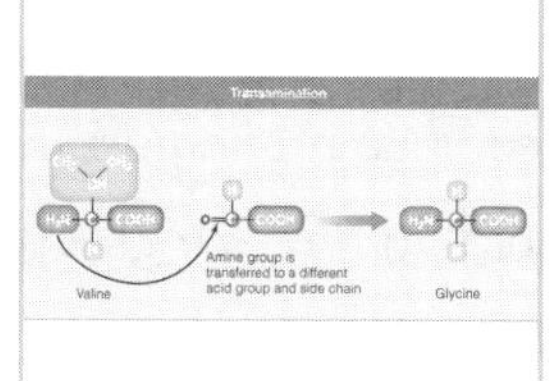

Figure 6.2
Transamination.

II. How Are Proteins Made? (p. 214)

a. Amino Acids Bond to Form a Variety of Peptides

b. Genes Regulate Amino Acid Bonding

c. Protein Turnover Involves Synthesis and Degradation

d. Protein Organization Determines Function

e. Protein Synthesis Can Be Limited by Missing Amino Acids

f. Protein Synthesis Can Be Enhanced by Mutual Supplementation

Key Terms: peptide bonds, gene expression, transcription, translation, limiting amino acid, incomplete proteins, complete proteins, mutual supplementation, complementary proteins

Instructor Tools: Chapter 6 PPT slides, Chapter 6 PRS Clicker Questions slide 1, TAs 124–129

Animation: *Protein Synthesis*

Images:

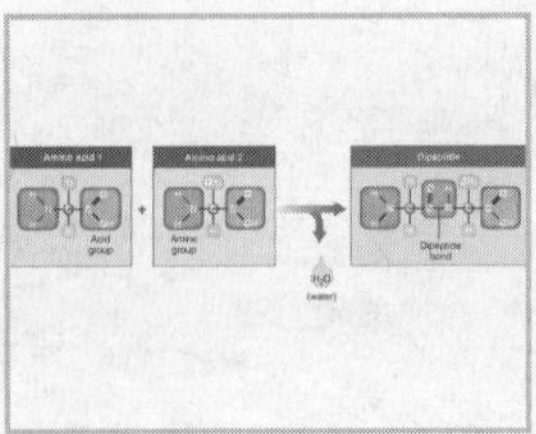

Figure 6.3
Amino acid bonding.

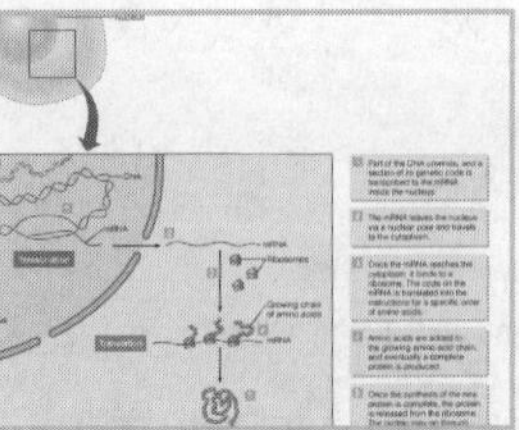

Figure 6.4
Gene expression.

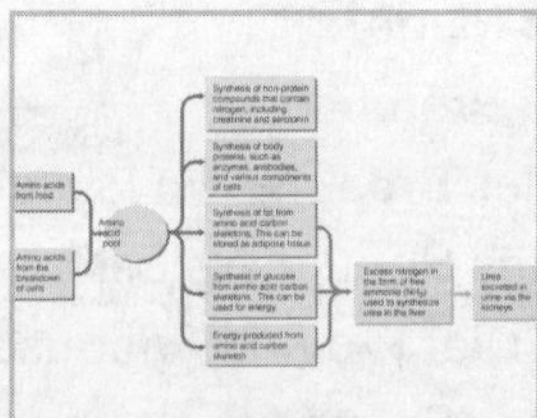

Figure 6.5
Protein turnover.

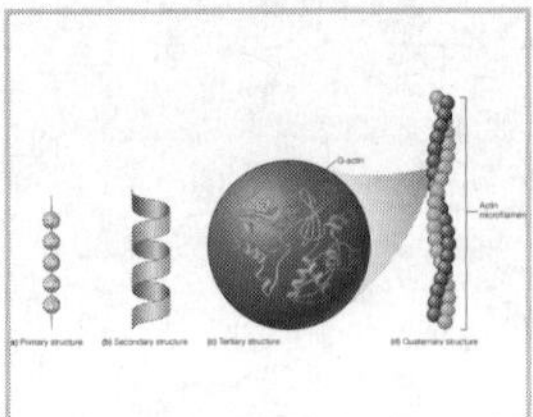

Figure 6.6
Levels of protein structure.

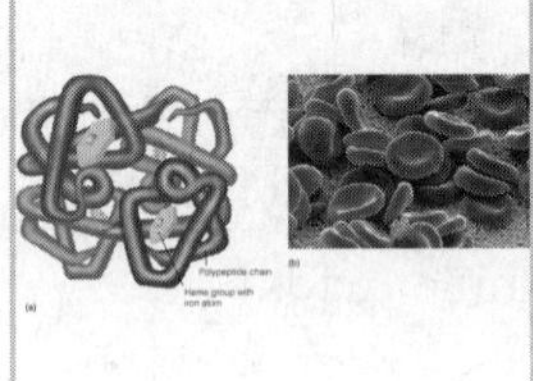

Figure 6.7
Protein shape determines function.

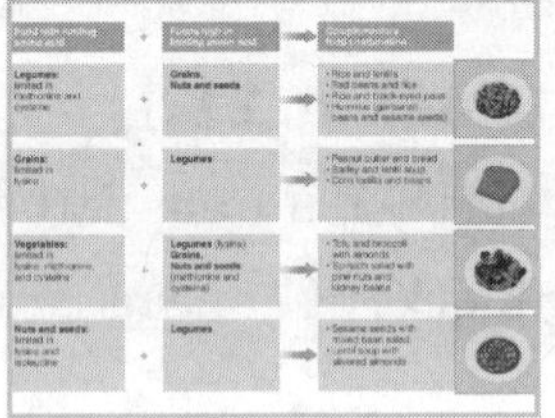

Figure 6.8
Complementary food combinations.

Activity:

The following demonstration illustrates the action of an enzyme and the loss of function when the enzyme is denatured.

Bring to class:

Prepared 2-3 cm Jello brand gelatin cubes (4-5 cubes per group)

Shallow dish or pan for each group

Fresh* and canned pineapple juice

*To prepare fresh pineapple juice, puree fresh pineapple in a blender. Strain the puree through cheesecloth to separate the pulp from the juice.

Give each student group several cubes of Jello in a shallow or dish or pan.

Give each student group a sample of either fresh or canned pineapple juice and instruct them to pour the juice over the Jello until the bottom of the dish or pan is covered.

Have students observe the Jello cubes for 30 minutes and note observations at 5 minute intervals.

The enzyme bromelin in the fresh pineapple juice will breakdown the collagen in the Jello. The canning process denatures bromelin, rendering the canned juice incapable of catalyzing the breakdown of gelatin.

III. Why Do We Need Proteins? (p. 220)

a. Proteins Contribute to Cell Growth, Repair, and Maintenance
b. Proteins Act as Enzymes and Hormones
c. Proteins Help Maintain Fluid and Electrolyte Balance
d. Proteins Help Maintain Acid-Base Balance
e. Proteins Help Maintain a Strong Immune System
f. Proteins Serve as an Energy Source

Key Terms: enzymes, edema, transport proteins, pH, acidosis, alkalosis, buffers, antibodies, deamination

Instructor Tools: Chapter 6 PPT slides, Chapter 6 PRS Clicker Questions slides 2–3, TAs 130–132

Animations: *Enzymes, Deamination/Transamination*

Images:

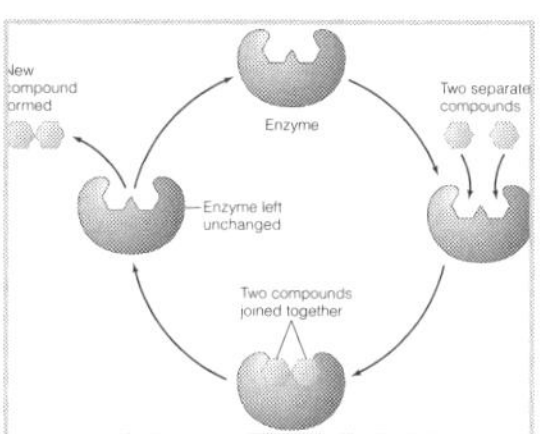

Figure 6.9
Proteins act as enzymes.

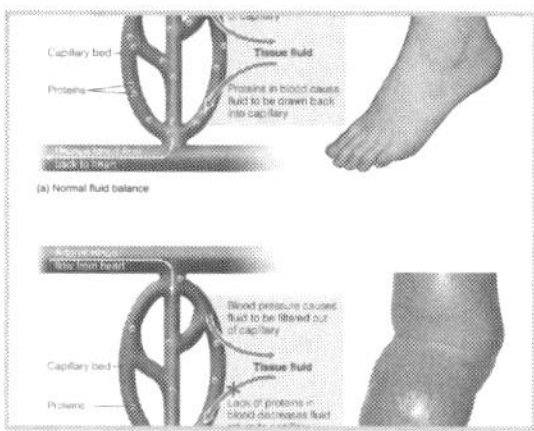

Figure 6.10
The role of proteins in maintaining fluid balance.

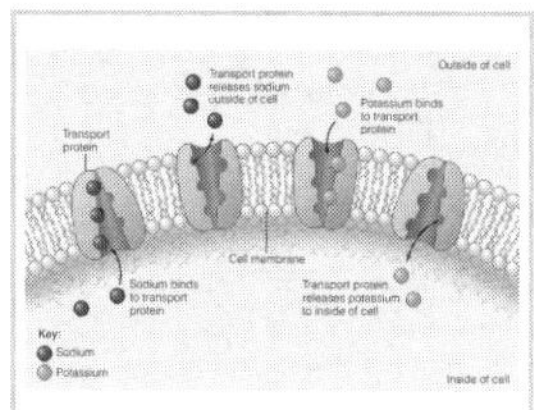

Figure 6.11
Transport proteins help maintain electrolyte balance.

IV. How Do Our Bodies Break Down Proteins? (p. 224)

a. Stomach Acids and Enzymes Break Proteins into Short Polypeptides
b. Enzymes in the Small Intestine Break Polypeptides into Single Amino Acids
c. Protein Digestibility Affect Protein Quality

Key Terms: pepsin, proteases, protein digestibility corrected amino acid score (PDCAAS)

Instructor Tools: Chapter 6 PPT slides, TA 133

Animations: *Protein Digestion, Protein Absorption*

Image:

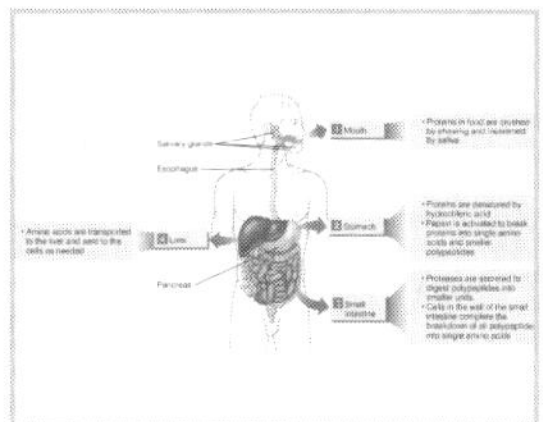

Figure 6.12
The process of protein digestion.

V. How Much Protein Should We Eat? (p. 226)

a. Nitrogen Balance Is a Method Used to Determine Protein Needs

b. Recommended Dietary Allowance (RDA) for Protein

c. Most Americans Meet or Exceed the RDA for Protein

d. Too Much Dietary Protein Can Be Harmful

e. Shopper's Guide: Good Food Sources of Protein

abc NEWS Lecture Launcher Video:

Atkins Diet

abc NEWS Video Discussion Questions:

1. Does eating fat make you fat? Explain.
2. Can eating fat make you thin? Explain.
3. Do you think the Food Guide Pyramid has contributed to weight gain? Explain.
4. Can eating carbohydrates make you fat? Explain.

Instructor Tools: Chapter 6 PPT slides, Chapter 6 PRS Clicker Questions slide 4, TAs 134, 139–142

Animation: *Nitrogen Balance*

Images:

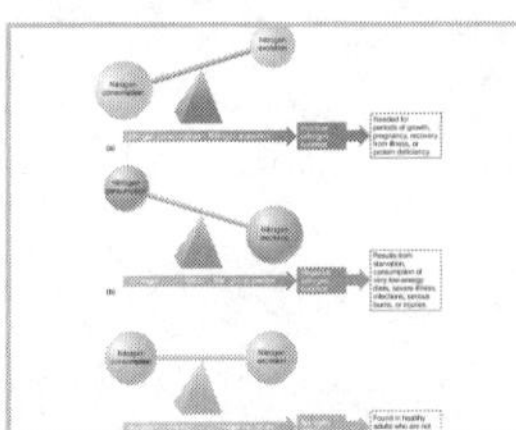

Figure 6.13
Nitrogen balance.

TABLE 6.2 Recommended Protein Intakes

Group	Protein Intake (g/kg body weight/day)*
Most adults†	0.8
Nonvegetarian endurance athletes‡	1.2 to 1.4
Nonvegetarian strength athletes‡	1.6 to 1.7
Vegetarian endurance athletes‡	1.3 to 1.5
Vegetarian strength athletes‡	1.7 to 1.8

*To convert body weight to kilograms, divide weight in pounds by 2.2.
Weight (lb)/2.2 = Weight (kg)
Weight (kg) × protein recommendation (g/kg body weight/day) = protein intake (g/day)
Sources: †Food and Nutrition Board, Institute of Medicine. 2005. *Dietary Reference Intakes for Energy, Carbohydrate, Fiber, Fat, Fatty Acids, Cholesterol, Protein, and Amino Acids (Macronutrients)*, pp. 465–608. Washington, DC: National Academies Press.
‡American College of Sports Medicine, American Dietetic Association, and Dietitians of Canada. 2001. Joint Position Statement. Nutrition and athletic performance. *Med. Sci. Sports Exerc.* 32:2130–2145.

Table 6.2
Recommended Protein Intakes

TABLE 6.3 Self-Reported Protein Intakes of Athletes

Sport Type	Gender	Protein Intake (g/kg body weight/day)	Protein Intake (% total kcal)
Football	M	1.5	15.0
Weightlifting	M	1.9	18.0
Soccer	M	2.2	14.4
Triathlon	M	2.0	13.0
Marathon running	M	2.0	14.5
Distance running	M	1.6	12.8
	F	1.1	14.1
Ultradistance running	M	1.4	16.7
	F	1.2	15.1
Bodybuilding	M	2.7–3.1	22.5–37.7
	F	1.9–2.7	22.6–35.8

Source: Adapted by permission from M. Manore and J. Thompson, 2000, *Sport Nutrition for Health and Performance*, page 118, Table 4.5. © 2000 by Melinda Manore and Janice Thompson. Reprinted with permission from Human Kinetics (Champaign, IL).

Table 6.3
Self-reported Protein Intakes of Athletes

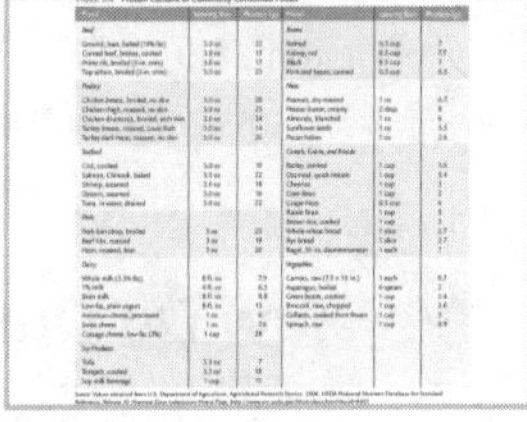

Table 6.4
Protein Content of Commonly Consumed Foods

Activity:

Instruct students to gather information on protein supplements marketed to body builders. Have students work in small groups to evaluate the value and safety of these supplements. Students should note how the cost of these supplements compares with the cost of food sources of protein.

VI. Can a Vegetarian Diet Provide Adequate Protein? (p. 234)

a. Types of Vegetarian Diets

b. Why Do People Become Vegetarians?

c. What Are the Challenges of a Vegetarian Diet?

d. Using the Vegetarian Food Guide Pyramid to Achieve the RDA for Protein

Key Terms: vegetarianism, mad cow disease, carcinogens

Instructor Tools: Chapter 6 PPT slides, Chapter 6 PRS Clicker Questions slide 5, TAs 135, 143–145

Images:

Table 6.5
Terms and Definitions of a Vegetarian Diet

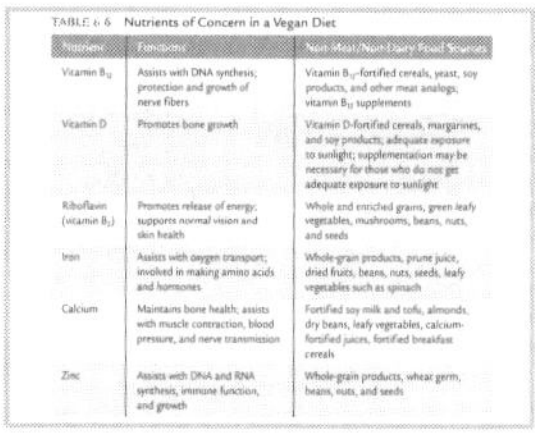

TABLE 6.6 Nutrients of Concern in a Vegan Diet

Nutrient	Functions	Non-Meat/Non-Dairy Food Sources
Vitamin B_{12}	Assists with DNA synthesis; protection and growth of nerve fibers	Vitamin B_{12}-fortified cereals, yeast, soy products, and other meat analogs; vitamin B_{12} supplements
Vitamin D	Promotes bone growth	Vitamin D-fortified cereals, margarines, and soy products; adequate exposure to sunlight; supplementation may be necessary for those who do not get adequate exposure to sunlight
Riboflavin (vitamin B_2)	Promotes release of energy; supports normal vision and skin health	Whole and enriched grains, green leafy vegetables, mushrooms, beans, nuts, and seeds
Iron	Assists with oxygen transport; involved in making amino acids and hormones	Whole-grain products, prune juice, dried fruits, beans, nuts, seeds, leafy vegetables such as spinach
Calcium	Maintains bone health; assists with muscle contraction, blood pressure, and nerve transmission	Fortified soy milk and tofu, almonds, dry beans, leafy vegetables, calcium-fortified juices, fortified breakfast cereals
Zinc	Assists with DNA and RNA synthesis, immune function, and growth	Whole-grain products, wheat germ, beans, nuts, and seeds

Table 6.6
Nutrients of Concern in a Vegan Diet

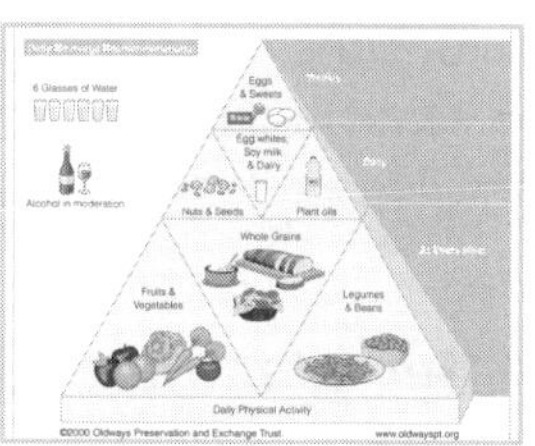

Figure 6.14
The Vegetarian Food Guide Pyramid.

Table 6.7
Food Groups and Recommended Serving Sizes for Vegetarians

Activities:

1. Using the Vegetarian Food Guide Pyramid in Figure 6.12b as a guide, have students work in small groups to plan a vegetarian menu that meets their RDA for protein. The Exchange System discussed in Chapter 2 can help determine the amount of protein in each food. You may want to assign different types of vegetarian diets to different groups—for example, a pescovegetarian, a lacto-ovo-vegetarian, and a vegan plan.

   Note: Because some of these plans are restrictive in their food choices, it may not be possible to include all food groups. Students should note which food groups are omitted in these plans.

2. Have students bring in either a main dish recipe that includes meat or a meatless main dish recipe to share with their classmates. Plan ahead so approximately half the recipes will be of each type. Instruct students to calculate the protein content of their recipe by using the food composition tables in the appendix. The total protein in the recipe should be divided by the number of servings to determine the amount of protein per serving. Compare the protein content of the dishes with meat and those without meat. Ask students to note which ingredients provide the most protein in these dishes.

VII. What Disorders Are Related to Protein Intake or Metabolism? (p. 242)

a. Protein-Energy Malnutrition Can Lead to Debility and Death
b. Disorders Related to Genetic Abnormalities

Key Terms: protein-energy malnutrition, marasmus, kwashiorkor, sickle cell anemia, cystic fibrosis

Instructor Tools: Chapter 6 PPT slides, TAs 136–137

Images:

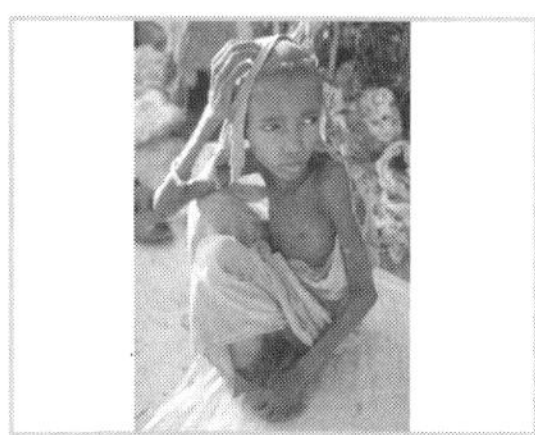

Figure 6.15a
Marasmus.

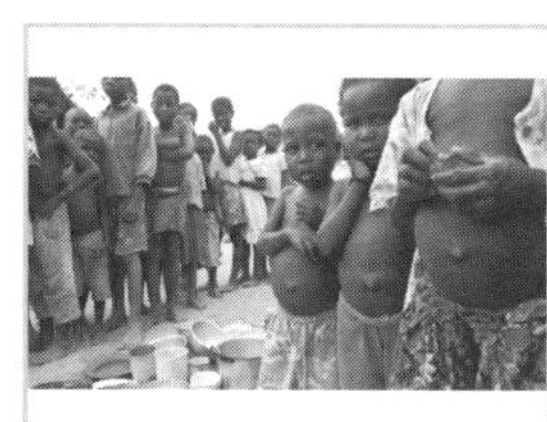

Figure 6.15b
Kwashiorkor.

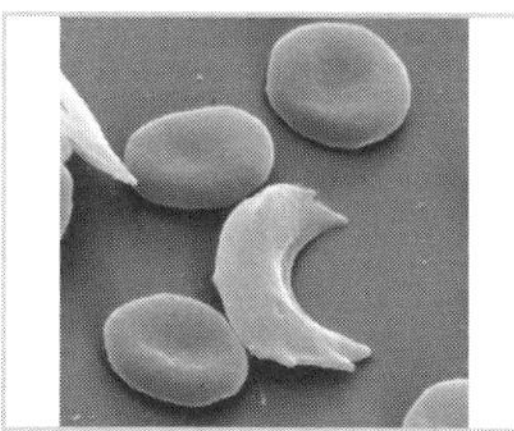

Figure 6.16
A sickled red blood cell.

Activity:

Have students research the issue of worldwide malnutrition by collecting newspaper and magazine articles or by searching the Internet. Discuss in class the areas in the world most affected by malnutrition, the consequences, and the efforts being made to solve it.

VIII. Additional Chapter 6 Instructor Tools

MyDietAnalysis Activity: Using the nutritional assessment previously completed, students should note the following:

1. How many grams of protein do you consume daily?
2. What percentage of your daily calories comes from protein?
3. Does your protein intake meet recommendations?
4. What three foods that you consumed that contained the highest amount of protein? How many grams of protein were in each food?
5. What changes can you make in your diet to more closely meet protein recommendations?

Nutrition Debate Activity: Instruct students to choose three meals and two snacks that are recommended on the Atkins Diet. These can be obtained from the recipe section of one of Atkins' books, from food labels on Atkins-approved prepared meals, or by going online to http://www.Atkins.com/recipes. Students should then:

1. Record the amount of protein each meal and snack provides.
2. Add up the total protein intake that this meal plan would provide.
3. Note how the protein intake for this plan compares with recommended protein intakes.

As an additional investigation, amount of fat, saturated fat, and carbohydrate can also be totaled for the day and compared with recommendations.

Printed TestBank: Pages 74–88 (TestGen Chapter 6)

MyDietAnalysis Online Assignments: Liz: High-Protein Diet; Theo: Diet and Macronutrients

Quiz Show PowerPoints: Chapter 6

In Depth: Vitamins and Minerals: Micronutrients with Macro Powers

Chapter at a Glance

I. Discovering the "Hidden" Nutrients
II. How Are Vitamins Classified?
III. How Are Minerals Classified?
IV. How Do Our Bodies Use Micronutrients?
V. Controversies in Micronutrient Metabolism

Visual Lecture Outline

I. Discovering the "Hidden" Nutrients (p. 253)

Key Term: micronutrients

Instructor Tools: In Depth: Vitamins and Minerals PPT slides, In Depth: Vitamins and Minerals PRS Clicker Questions slide 1

II. How Are Vitamins Classified? (p. 253)

a. Fat-Soluble Vitamins

b. Water-Soluble Vitamins

Key Terms: vitamins, fat-soluble vitamins, megadoses, water-soluble vitamins

Instructor Tools: In Depth: Vitamins and Minerals PPT slides, In Depth: Vitamins and Minerals PRS Clicker Questions slide 2, TAs 147–151

Images:

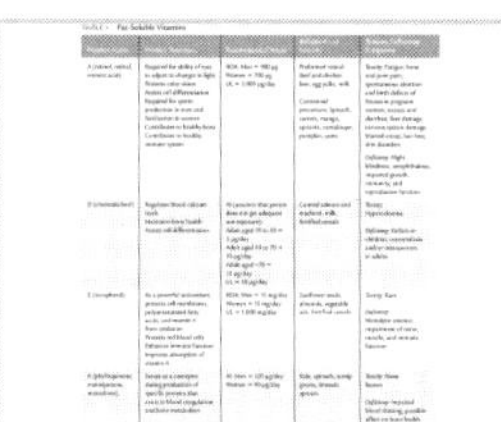

Table 1
Fat-Soluble Vitamins

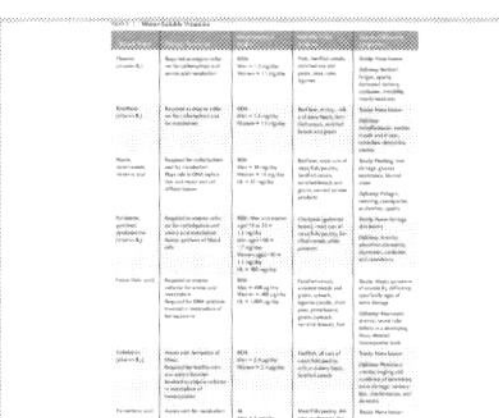

Table 2a
Water-Soluble Vitamins

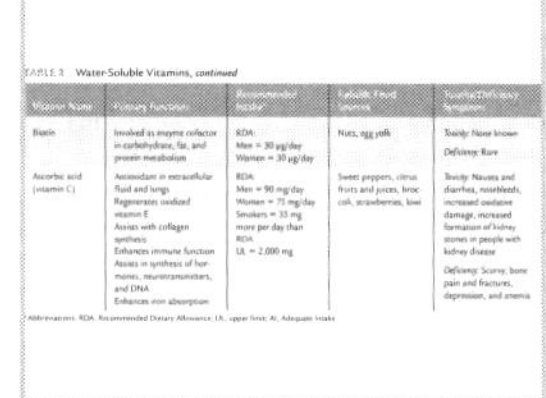

Table 2b
Water-Soluble Vitamins, *continued*

III. How Are Minerals Classified? (p. 255)

a. Major Minerals

b. Trace Minerals

c. Same Mineral, Different Forms

Key Terms: minerals, major minerals, trace minerals

Instructor Tools: In Depth: Vitamins and Minerals PPT slides, In Depth: Vitamins and Minerals PRS Clicker Questions slides 3–4, TAs 152–156

Images:

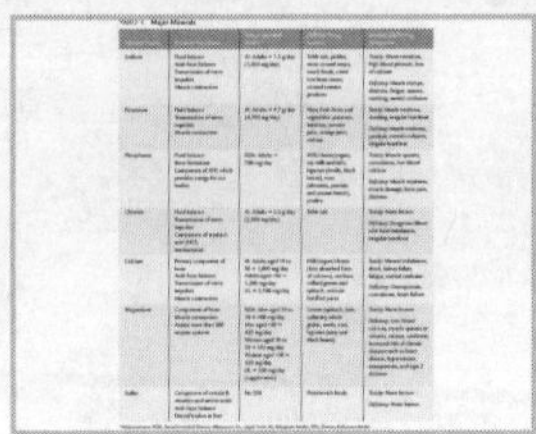

Table 3
Major Minerals

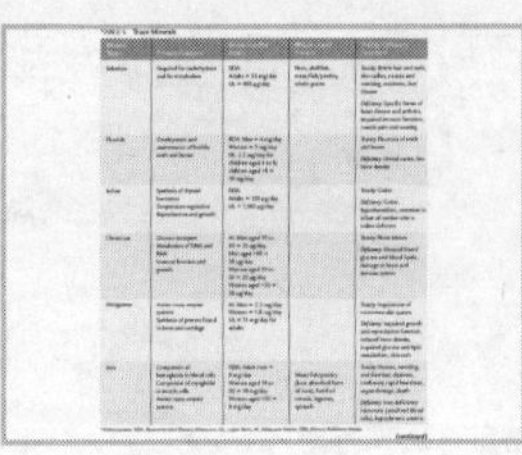

Table 4a
Trace Minerals

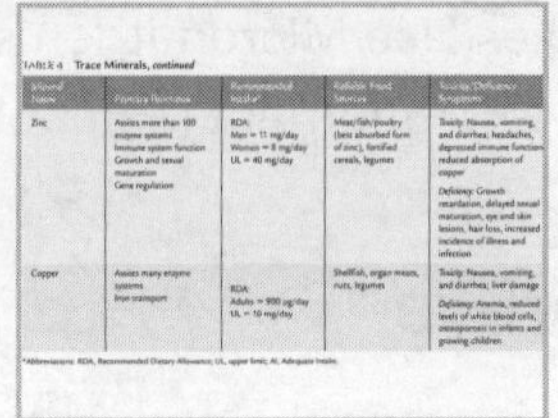

Table 4b
Trace Minerals, *continued*

IV. How Do Our Bodies Use Micronutrients? (p. 260)

a. What We Eat Differs from What We Absorb

b. What We Eat Differs from What Our Cells Use

Key Terms: heme iron, non-heme iron

Instructor Tools: In Depth: Vitamins and Minerals PPT slides, In Depth: Vitamins and Minerals PRS Clicker Questions slide 5

V. Controversies in Micronutrient Metabolism (p. 262)

a. Are Supplements Healthful Sources of Micronutrients?

b. Can Micronutrients Really Prevent or Treat Disease?

c. Do More Essential Micronutrients Exist?

Instructor Tools: In Depth: Vitamins and Minerals PPT slides

Activities:

1. Ask students to bring a label from a vitamin/mineral supplement to class. This can be obtained from an actual supplement bottle or from an internet investigation of a particular supplement. Have students work in groups to evaluate the contents of each supplement. The evaluation should include:
   a. Does the supplement contain all vitamins and minerals with established RDIs? If not, which nutrients are missing?
   b. Are most nutrients present at or near 100% of the RDIs? Note vitamins or minerals that are present in low or extremely high amounts.
   c. Note the form (or forms) of the vitamins and minerals present.

A class discussion could follow this activity to further explore how the form of the nutrient might affect absorption and what the advantages and disadvantages of these supplements might be.

2. Ask students to bring vitamin/mineral supplements to class. Add vinegar to small, clear cups and add one supplement to each cup. Let the supplements sit in the cups for 15 to 30 minutes. Swirl each cup every 5 minutes. Record observations. Discuss the implications of supplements that haven't dissolved at the end of the testing period.

VI. Additional In Depth: Vitamins and Minerals Instructor Tools

MyDietAnalysis Activity: Using the nutritional assessment previously completed, have students note their top source of the following nutrients:

- vitamin C
- folate
- vitamin B_{12}
- thiamin
- riboflavin
- vitamin D
- iron
- calcium

Discuss with the class the importance of a varied diet.

Printed TestBank: Pages 89–92 (TestGen In Depth: Vitamins and Minerals)

Notes

Nutrients Involved in Fluid and Electrolyte Balance 7

Chapter at a Glance

I. What Are Fluids and Electrolytes, and What Are their Functions?
II. How Do Our Bodies Maintain Fluid Balance?
III. A Profile of Nutrients Involved in Hydration and Neuromuscular Function
IV. What Disorders Are Related to Fluid and Electrolyte Imbalances?

Visual Lecture Outline

I. What Are Fluids and Electrolytes, and What Are their Functions? (p. 266)

a. Body Fluid Is the Liquid Portion of Our Cells and Tissues
b. Body Fluid Is Composed of Water and Dissolved Substances Called Electrolytes
c. Fluids Serve Many Critical Functions
d. Electrolytes Support Many Body Functions

Key Terms: fluid, intracellular fluid, extracellular fluid, electrolyte, ion, solvent, blood volume, osmosis

Instructor Tools: Chapter 7 PPT slides, Chapter 7 PRS Clicker Questions slides 1–2, TAs 157–162

Animation: *Intracellular and Extracellular Fluid*

Images:

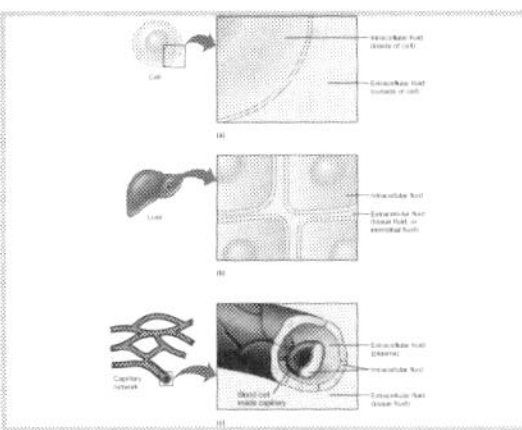

Figure 7.1
The components of body fluid.

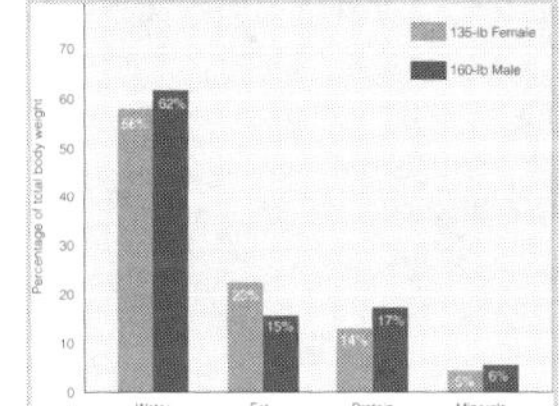

Figure 7.2
Body composition of an average adult male and female.

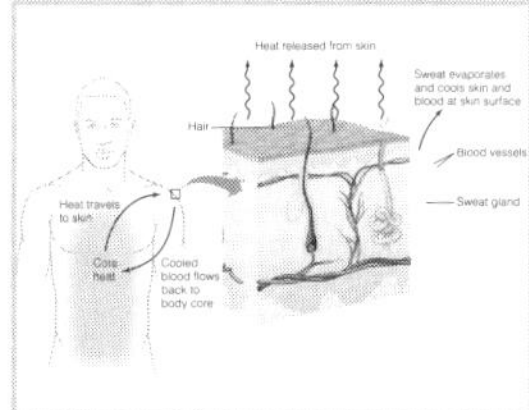

Figure 7.3
Evaporative cooling occurs when heat is transported from the body core through the bloodstream to the surface of the skin.

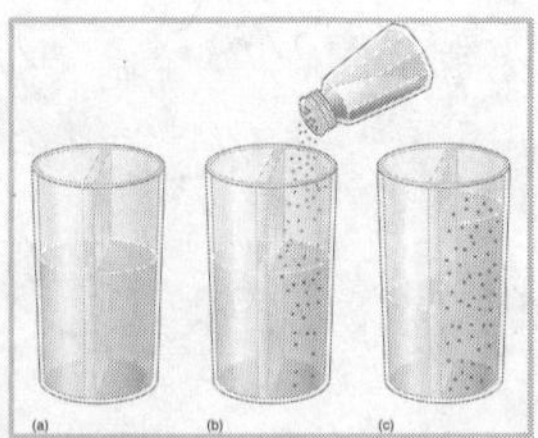

Figure 7.4
Osmosis.

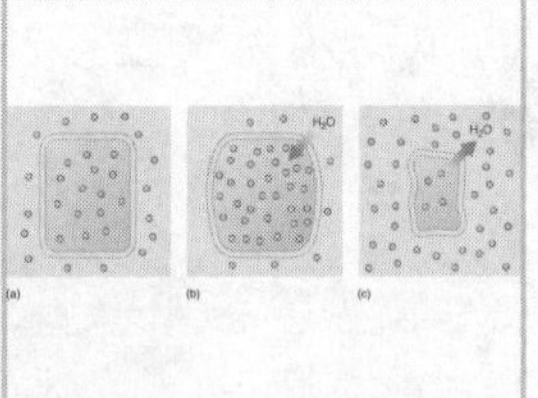

Figure 7.5
The health of our body's cells depends on maintaining the proper balance of fluids and electrolytes on either side of the cell membrane.

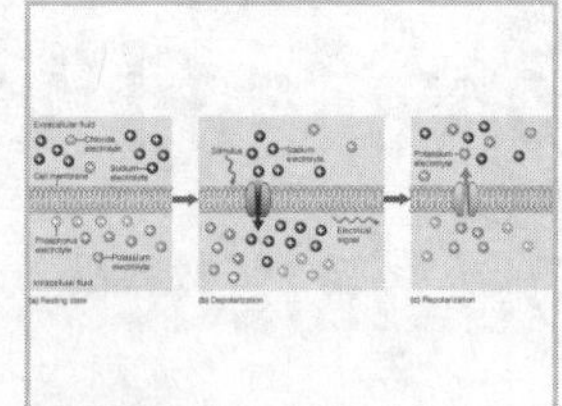

Figure 7.6
The role of electrolytes in conduction of a nerve impulse.

Activities:

1. To demonstrate the movement of water into cells, place a piece of limp celery into a container of water with red food coloring added. Examine the celery every 30 minutes during class to check for firmness and to observe the location of the dye.
2. For a quick and easy demonstration of how water evaporation off the skin's surface can cool the body, ask students to place a wet hand and a dry hand in front of a fan. After about 30 to 60 seconds, ask students which hand feels cooler.

II. How Do Our Bodies Maintain Fluid Balance? (p. 272)

a. Our Thirst Mechanism Prompts Us to Drink Fluids
b. We Gain Fluids by Consuming Beverages and Foods and Through Metabolism
c. We Lose Fluids Through Urine, Sweat, Evaporation, Exhalation, and Feces

Key Terms: thirst mechanism, metabolic water, sensible water loss, insensible water loss, diuretic

Instructor Tools: Chapter 7 PPT slides, Chapter 7 PRS Clicker Questions slide 3, TA 163

Animations: *Water Balance, Electrolytes in Water Balance*

Image:

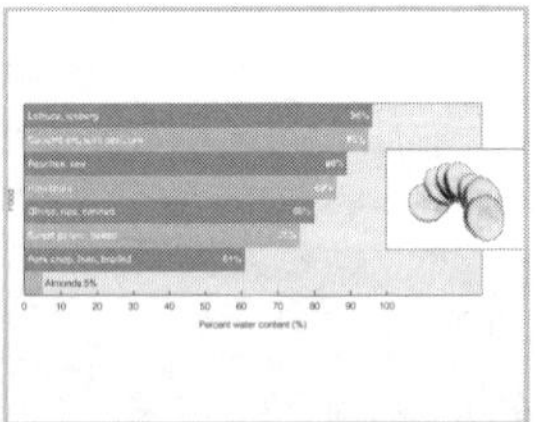

Figure 7.7
Water content of different foods.

Activity:

For a quick and easy demonstration of how water evaporation off the skin's surface can cool the body, ask students to place a wet hand and a dry hand in front of a fan. After about 30 to 60 seconds, ask students which hand feels cooler.

III. A Profile of Nutrients Involved in Hydration and Neuromuscular Function (p. 276)

a. Water

b. Sodium

c. Shopper's Guide: Sources of Sodium

d. Potassium

e. Shopper's Guide: Good Food sources of Potassium

f. Chloride

g. Phosphorus

abc NEWS **Lecture Launcher Video:**

Bottled Water

abc NEWS **Video Discussion Questions:**

1. What are potential hazards in tap water?
2. Do you have a preference for tap water or bottled water? Which one do you prefer and why?
3. How effective do you believe marketing is in influencing your preference for foods and beverages?

Key Terms: hypernatremia, hyponatremia, hyperkalemia, hypokalemia, phytic acid, dehydration

Instructor Tools: Chapter 7 PPT slides, TAs 164–166, 169–171

Images:

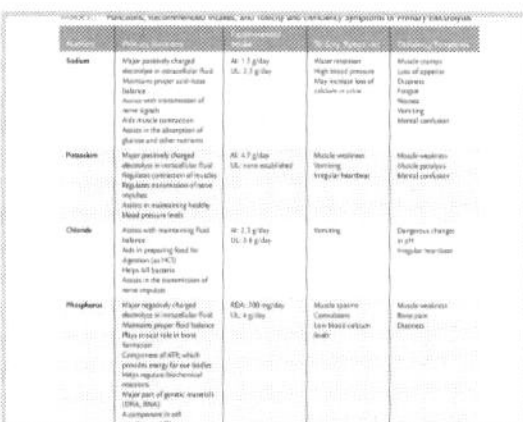

Table 7.1
Functions, Recommended Intakes, and Toxicity and Deficiency Symptoms of Primary Electrolytes

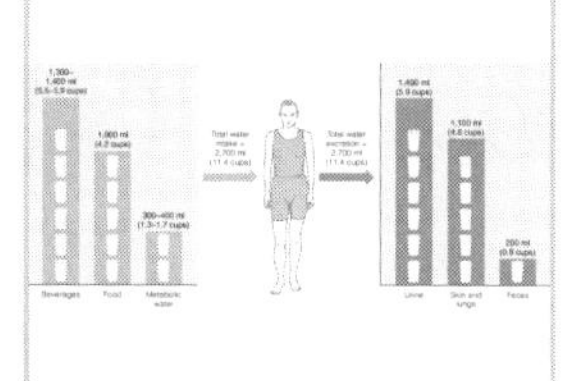

Figure 7.8
Amount and sources of water intake and output for a woman expending 2,500 kcal per day.

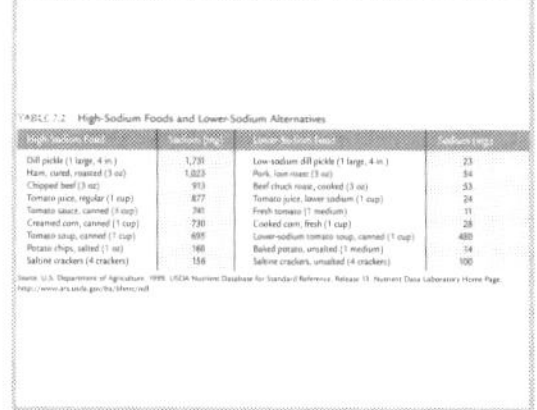

Table 7.2
High-Sodium Foods and Lower-Sodium Alternatives

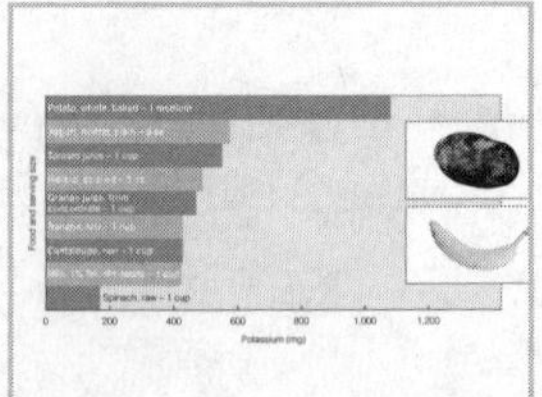

Figure 7.9
Common food sources of potassium.

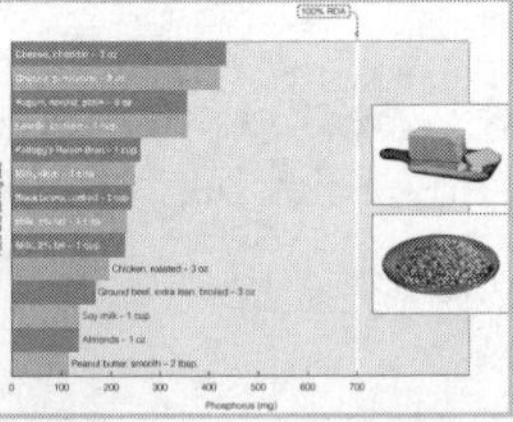

Figure 7.10
Common food sources of phosphorus.

Activity:

Ask for volunteers to prepare at home one of their favorite vegetables without adding salt or another sodium additive and to bring it to class. Ask other students to volunteer to bring in several different salt substitutes. Divide the prepared vegetables into portions. Leave some vegetables unflavored. Add the salt substitutes to others. Allow students to sample the various flavored and unflavored vegetables.

IV. What Disorders Are Related to Fluid and Electrolyte Imbalances? (p. 289)

a. Dehydration
b. Heat Stroke
c. Water Intoxication
d. Hypertension
e. Neuropsychiatric disorders
f. Muscle Disorders
g. Contribution of Fluids to Obesity

Key Terms: dehydration, heat stroke, overhydration, hypertension, seizures, muscle cramps

Instructor Tools: Chapter 7 PPT slides, Chapter 7 PRS Clicker Questions slides 4–6, TAs 167–168, 172

Images:

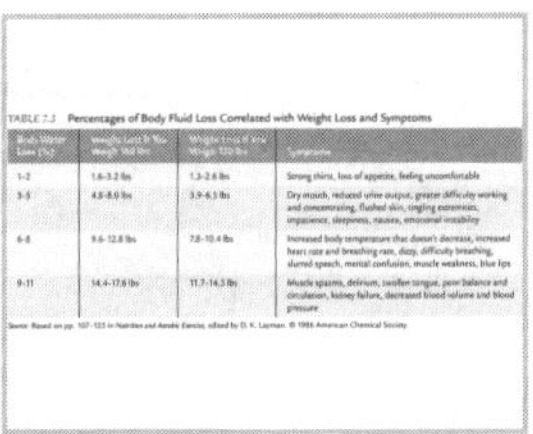

TABLE 7.3 Percentages of Body Fluid Loss Correlated with Weight Loss and Symptoms

Body Water Loss (%)	Weight Lost If You Weigh 160 lbs	Weight Loss If You Weigh 130 lbs	Symptoms
1–2	1.6–3.2 lbs	1.3–2.6 lbs	Strong thirst, loss of appetite, feeling uncomfortable
3–5	4.8–8.0 lbs	3.9–6.5 lbs	Dry mouth, reduced urine output, greater difficulty working and concentrating, flushed skin, tingling extremities, impatience, sleepiness, nausea, emotional instability
6–8	9.6–12.8 lbs	7.8–10.4 lbs	Increased body temperature that doesn't decrease, increased heart rate and breathing rate, dizzy, difficulty breathing, slurred speech, mental confusion, muscle weakness, blue lips
9–11	14.4–17.6 lbs	11.7–14.3 lbs	Muscle spasms, delirium, swollen tongue, poor balance and circulation, kidney failure, decreased blood volume and blood pressure

Source: Based on pp. 107–123 in Nutrition and Aerobic Exercise, edited by D. K. Layman. © 1986 American Chemical Society.

Table 7.3
Percentages of Body Fluid Loss Correlated with Weight Loss and Symptoms

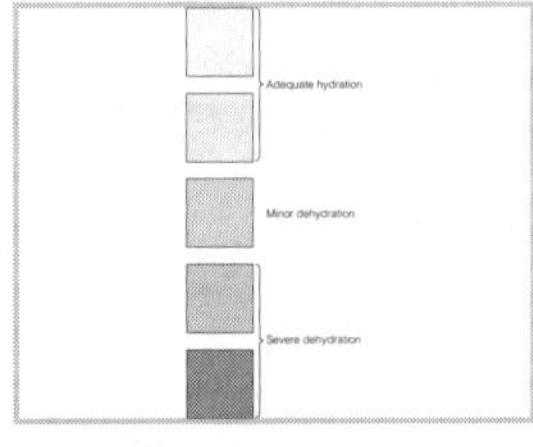

Figure 7.11
Urine color chart.

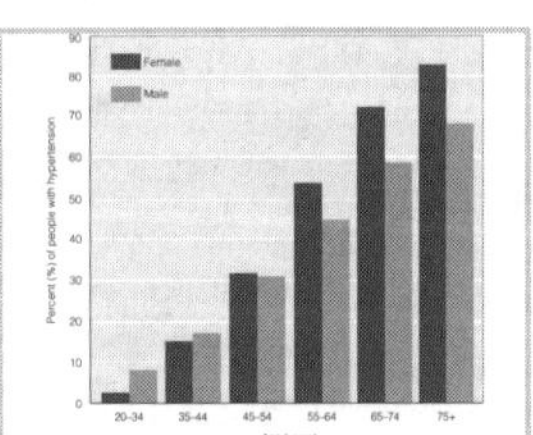

Figure 7.12
Hypertension is one of the major chronic diseases in the United States.

V. Additional Chapter 7 Instructor Tools

MyDietAnalysis Activity: Using the nutritional assessment previously completed, students should note the following:

1. How many milligrams of sodium do you consume daily?
2. How does your sodium intake compare to recommendations?
3. What three foods that you consumed contained the highest amount of sodium? How many milligrams of sodium were in each food?
4. How many milligrams of potassium do you consume daily?
5. How does your potassium intake compare to recommendations?
6. How much water do you consume daily?
7. How does your water intake compare to recommendations?

Nutrition Debate Activity: Ask each student to research a sports beverage that is currently available. Have students bring to class the Nutrition Facts Panel from the beverage they have investigated. Compile a list for each beverage that includes the following information (for a 12-ounce serving):

1. total calories in the beverage
2. grams of carbohydrate in the beverage
3. grams of protein in the beverage
4. milligrams of sodium in the beverage
5. milligrams of potassium in the beverage
6. Discuss any claims made by the manufacturers of these sports drinks and whether or not such claims are valid.

Printed TestBank: Pages 93–106 (TestGen Chapter 7)

Quiz Show PowerPoints: Chapter 7

Notes

Nutrients Involved in Antioxidant Function

8

Chapter at a Glance

I. What Are Antioxidants, and How Do Our Bodies Use Them?
II. A Profile of Nutrients That Function as Antioxidants
III. What Disorders Are Related to Free Radical Damage?

Visual Lecture Outline

I. What Are Antioxidants, and How Do Our Bodies Use Them? (p. 304)

a. Oxidation Is a Chemical Reaction in Which Atoms Lose Electrons
b. Oxidation Sometimes Results in the Formation of Free Radicals
c. Free Radicals Can Destabilize Other Molecules and Damage Our Cells
d. Antioxidants Work by Stabilizing Free Radicals or Opposing Oxidation

Key Terms: antioxidant, atom, nucleus, electron, oxidation, free radical, cofactor

Instructor Tools: Chapter 8 PPT slides, Chapter 8 PRS Clicker Questions slides 1–2, TAs 174–178

Animation: *Free Radical Formation*

Images:

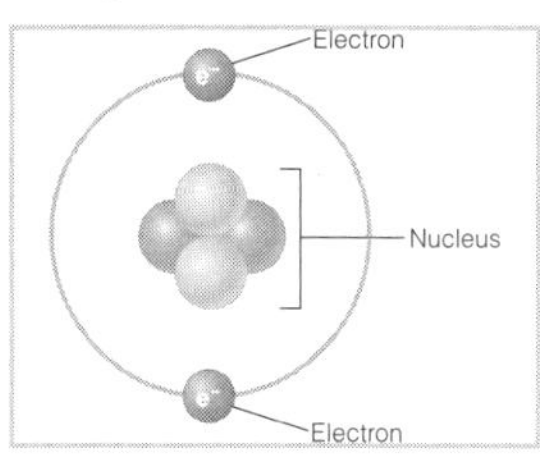

Figure 8.1
An atom consists of a central nucleus and orbiting electrons.

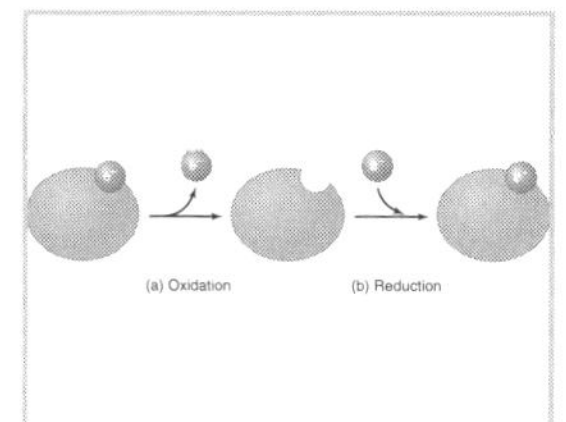

Figure 8.2
The exchange reaction.

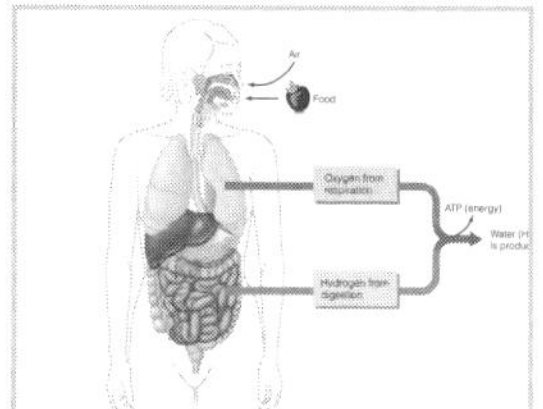
Figure 8.3
Oxygen and hydrogen exchange reactions during metabolism produce ATP and water.

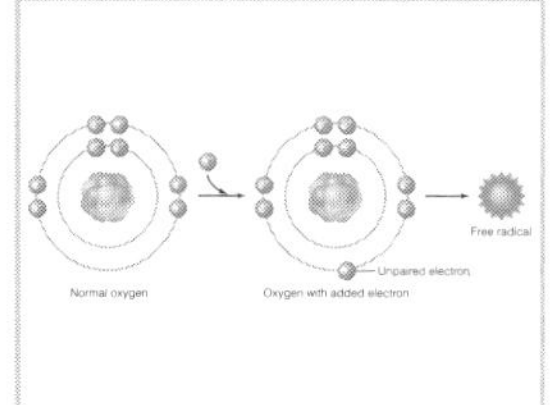
Figure 8.4
Formation of a free radical.

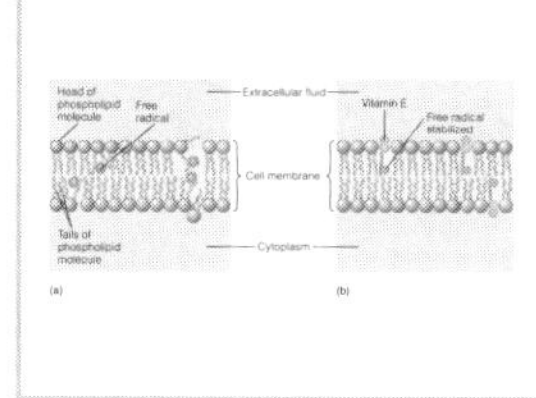
Figure 8.5
The formation of free radicals in the lipid portion of our cell membranes and stabilization by vitamin E.

II. A Profile of Nutrients That Function as Antioxidants (p. 308)

a. Vitamin E

b. Shopper's Guide: Good Food Sources of Vitamin E

c. Vitamin C

d. Shopper's Guide: Good Food Sources of Vitamin C

e. Beta-Carotene

f. Shopper's Guide: Good Food Sources of Beta-Carotene

g. Vitamin A

h. Selenium

i. Copper, Iron, Zinc, and Manganese Assist in Antioxidant Function

Key Terms: tocotrienol, tocopherol, collagen, megadose, prooxidant, provitamin, carotenoids, retinol, retinal, retinoic acid, retina, opsin, rhodopsin, cell differentiation, night blindness, Keshan disease

Instructor Tools: Chapter 8 PPT slides, Chapter 8 PRS Clicker Questions slides 3–5, TAs 179–187, 194–195

Animations: *Vitamin A and the Visual Cycle, Vitamin A and the Epithelial Tissue*

Images:

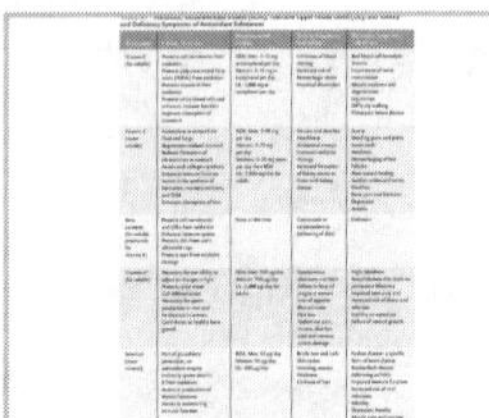

Table 8.1
Functions, RDAs, ULs, and Toxicity and Deficiency Symptoms of Antioxidant Substances

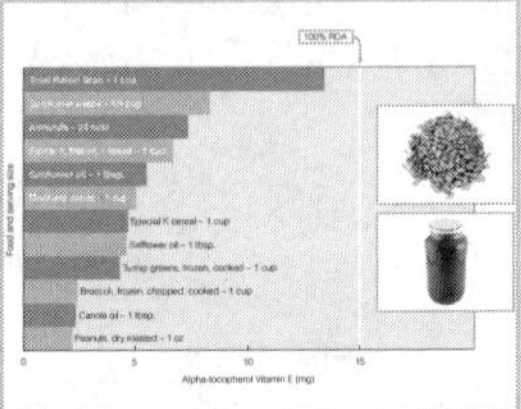

Figure 8.6
Common food sources of vitamin E.

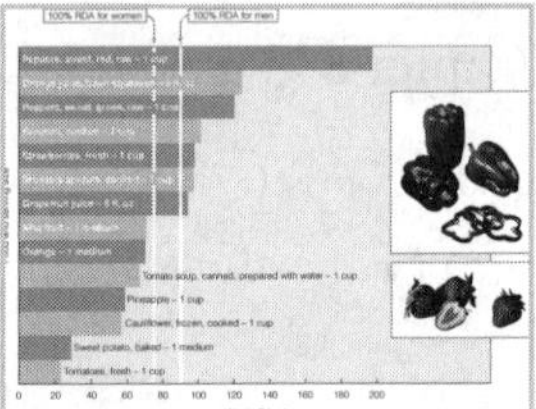

Figure 8.7
Common food sources of vitamin C.

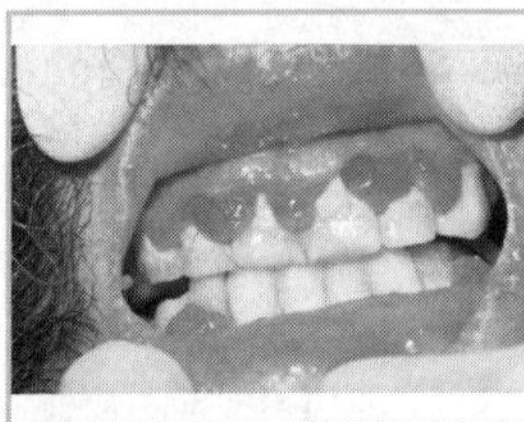

Figure 8.8
Bleeding gums from scurvy.

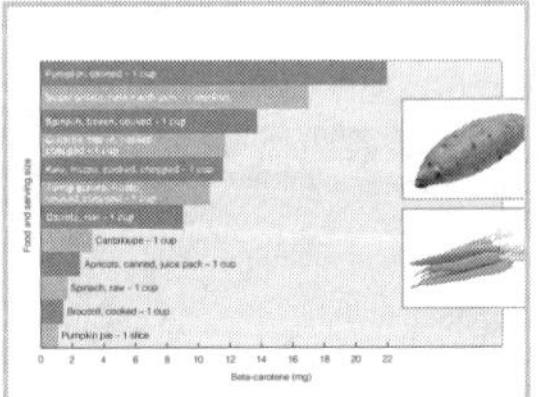

Figure 8.9
Common food sources of beta-carotene.

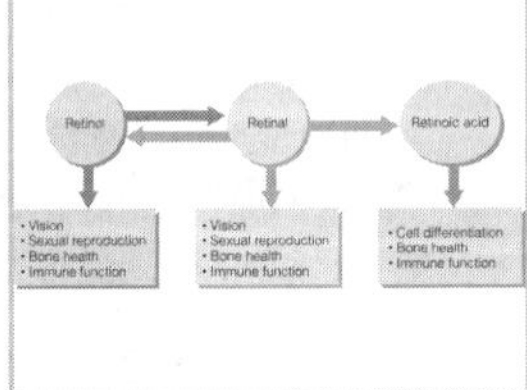

Figure 8.10
The three active forms of vitamin A in our bodies are retinol, retinal, and retinoic acid.

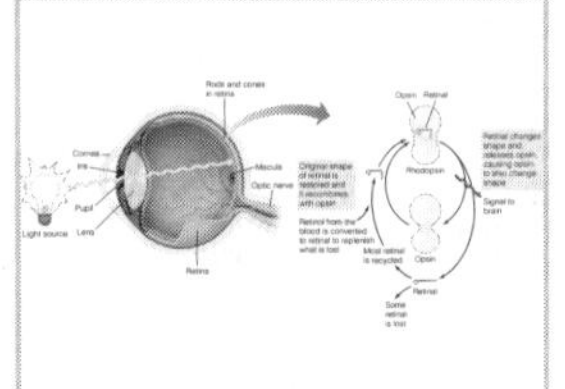

Figure 8.11
Vitamin A is necessary to maintain healthy vision.

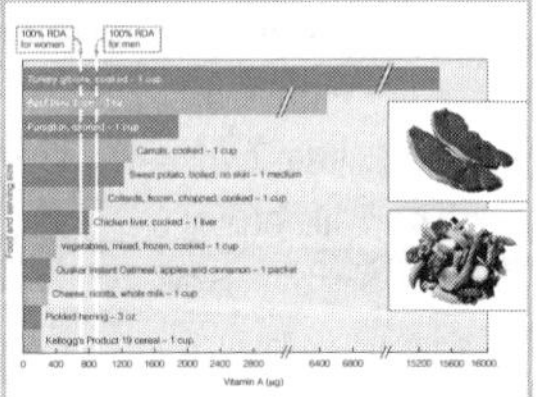

Figure 8.12
Common food sources of vitamin A.

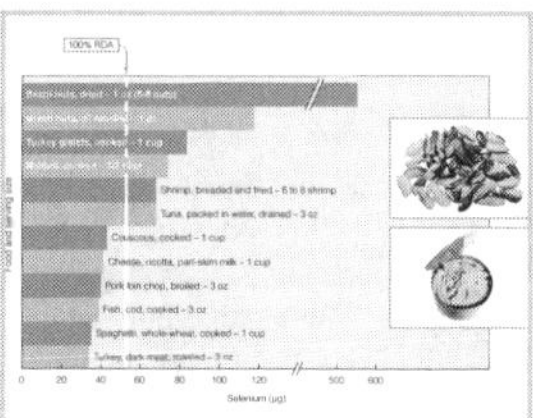
Figure 8.13
Common food sources of selenium.

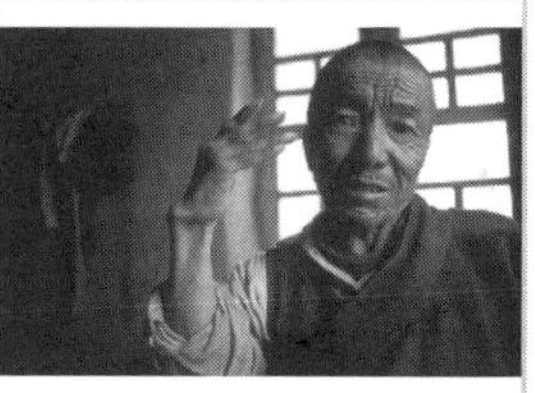
Figure 8.14
Selenium deficiency can lead to deforming arthritis called Kashin-Beck disease.

Activities:

1. To help students learn the nutrients discussed in this chapter, their functions, and their food sources, start by asking a student to name one nutrient. Then ask the next student to add a piece of information about that nutrient. Continue until you get four or five items of information about that nutrient. The next student names another nutrient. Repeat in this manner until all nutrients covered in this chapter have been reviewed.
2. Processed foods are often low in antioxidants. Ask students to choose a canned soup or frozen dinner to investigate. Have them read the nutrition label to find out how much vitamin A and C is in a serving. Students should share their findings with the class. Discuss the implications of a diet high in processed food.

III. What Disorders Are Related to Free Radical Damage? (p. 327)

a. Cancer
b. Cardiovascular Disease
c. Vision Impairment and Other Results of Aging

abc NEWS Lecture Launcher Video:

Tobacco Addiction

abc NEWS Video Discussion Questions:

1. If you have ever smoked or know someone who has smoked and successfully quit, what types of techniques were used to aid in quitting? Can you think of additional helpful suggestions to aid in quitting?
2. Do you believe the physical addiction or the psychological addiction is more difficult to overcome when quitting smoking? Give reasons to support your opinion.
3. According to the Surgeon General, adolescents are most likely to try smoking for the first time between the ages of 11 and 15. What types of techniques could be used to decrease the likelihood that these adolescents will begin smoking?

Key Terms: cancer, tumor, carcinogen, macular degeneration, cataract

Instructor Tools: Chapter 8 PPT slides, Chapter 8 PRS Clicker Questions slide 6, TAs 188–193

Images:

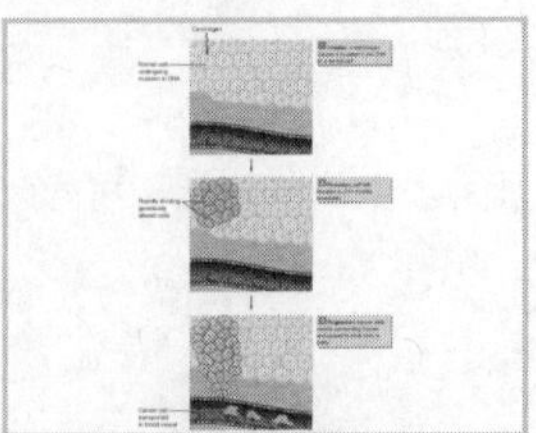

Figure 8.15
Cancer cells develop as a result of a genetic mutation in the DNA of a normal cell.

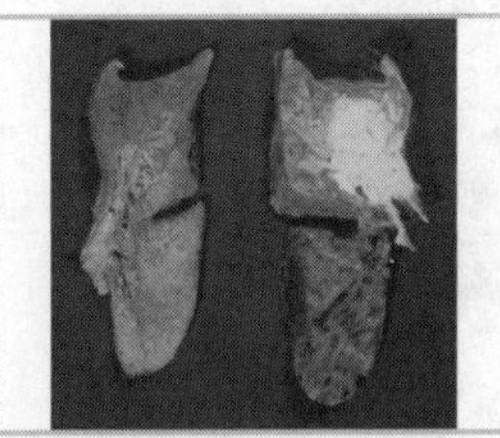

Figure 8.16
(a) A normal, healthy lung, (b) the lung of a smoker.

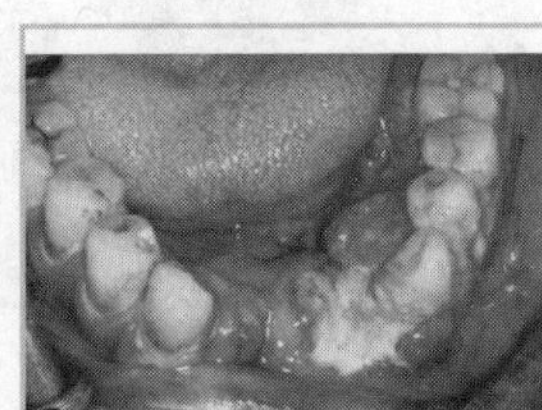

Figure 8.17a
Effects of tobacco use.
(a) mouth cancer.

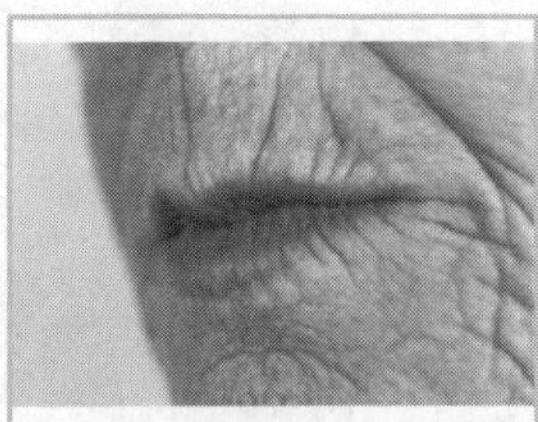

Figure 8.17b
Effects of tobacco use.
(b) premature wrinkling of the skin around the mouth.

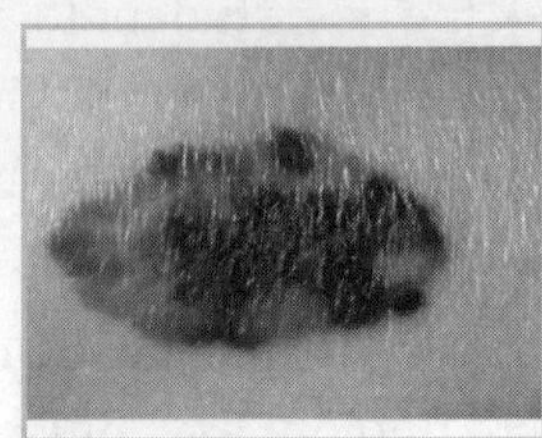

Figure 8.18
A lesion associated with malignant melanoma.

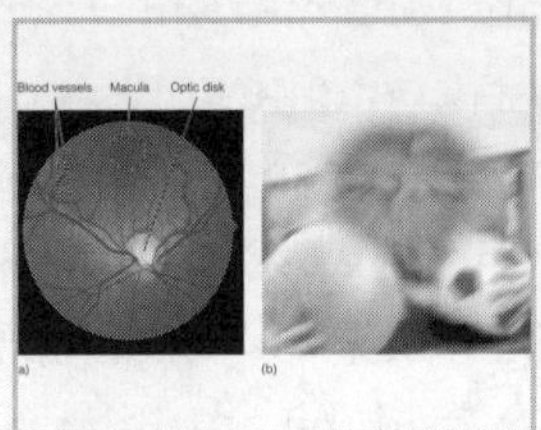

Figure 8.19
Macular degeneration.

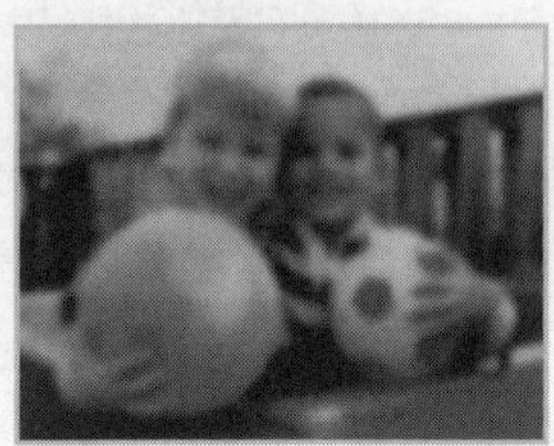

Figure 8.20
Cataracts can impair vision across the entire visual field.

IV. Additional Chapter 8 Instructor Tools

MyDietAnalysis Activity: Using the nutritional assessment previously completed, students should note the following:

1. What is your daily intake of:
   - vitamin E?
   - vitamin C?
   - vitamin A?
   - selenium?
2. How does your intake of these nutrients compare with recommendations?
3. What changes can you make in your diet to more closely meet recommendations?

Nutrition Debate Activity: Have students research vitamin/mineral supplements on the Internet and choose one to evaluate. Ask each student to evaluate the supplement using the six criteria suggested on p. 346 in the text. Students can then share their evaluations with the class.

Printed TestBank: Pages 107–122 (TestGen Chapter 8)

Quiz Show PowerPoints: Chapter 8

In Depth: Phytochemicals and Functional Foods

Chapter at a Glance

I. What Are Phytochemicals?
II. What Are Functional Foods?

Visual Lecture Outline

I. What Are Phytochemicals? (p. 351)

a. How Do Phytochemicals Reduce Our Risk of Disease?

b. Is There an RDA for Phytochemicals?

Key Terms: phytochemicals, diseases of aging, metabolites

Instructor Tools: In Depth: Phytochemicals and Functional Foods PPT slides, In Depth: Phytochemicals and Functional Foods PRS Clicker Questions slide 1, TA 200–201

Image:

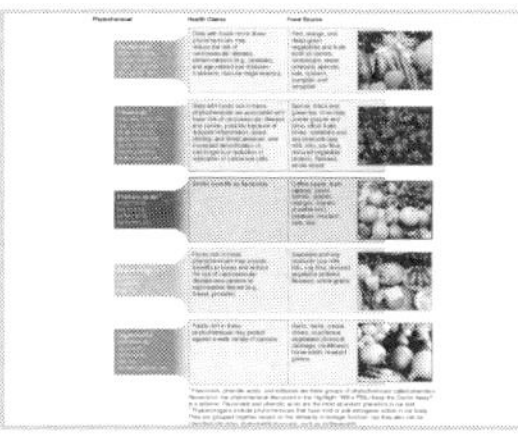

Figure 1
Health claims and food sources of phytochemicals.

Activity:

Have students work in groups and give them each one of the following meals to improve:

Breakfast: bagel and coffee

Lunch: cheese burger and diet soda

Dinner: pasta with sauce and diet soda

For each meal, ask students to suggest ways to increase intake of phytochemicals by adding food items to the meal, but without changing the given food items.

II. What Are Functional Foods (p. 354)

a. Are Functional Foods Safe?

b. Are Functional Foods Effective?

c. Are You Ready to Choose Functional Foods?

Key Terms: probiotics, prebiotics

Instructor Tools: In Depth: Phytochemicals and Functional Foods PPT slides, In Depth: Phytochemicals and Functional Foods PRS Clicker Questions slides 2–4

Activity:

Have students do a Web search or a search in a supermarket for a "functional" food. Ask students to analyze whether or not they believe the health claim of the manufacturer is a valid one. Discuss in class what type of evidence is used to support the health claims for the various products.

III. Additional In Depth: Phytochemicals and Functional Foods Instructor Tools

MyDietAnalysis Activity: Using the 3-day nutrition journal previously completed, have students note which foods in their journal contained phytochemicals. To help them with this activity Figure 1 on page 352 can be used.

Printed TestBank: Pages 123–126 (TestGen In Depth: Phytochemicals and Functional Foods)

Nutrients Involved in Bone Health

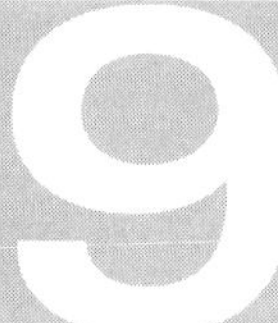

Chapter at a Glance

I. How Do Our Bodies Maintain Bone Health?
II. How Do We Assess Bone Health?
III. A Profile of Nutrients That Maintain Bone Health
IV. Osteoporosis Is a Disorder Resulting from Poor Bone Health

Visual Lecture Outline

I. How Do Our Bodies Maintain Bone Health? (p. 362)

a. Bone Composition and Structure Provide Strength and Flexibility

b. The Constant Activity of Bone Tissue Promotes Bone Health

Key Terms: collagen, cortical bone (compact bone), trabecular bone (spongy or cancellous bone), bone density, remodeling, resorption, osteoclasts, osteoblasts

Instructor Tools: Chapter 9 PPT slides, Chapter 9 PRS Clicker Questions slide 1, TAs 202–204, 220

Images:

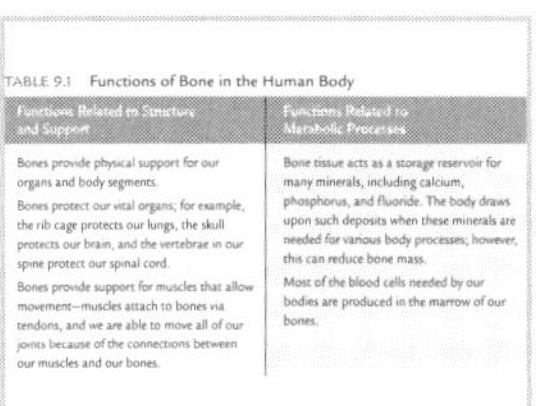

TABLE 9.1 Functions of Bone in the Human Body

Functions Related to Structure and Support	Functions Related to Metabolic Processes
Bones provide physical support for our organs and body segments.	Bone tissue acts as a storage reservoir for many minerals, including calcium, phosphorus, and fluoride. The body draws upon such deposits when these minerals are needed for various body processes; however, this can reduce bone mass.
Bones protect our vital organs; for example, the rib cage protects our lungs, the skull protects our brain, and the vertebrae in our spine protect our spinal cord.	Most of the blood cells needed by our bodies are produced in the marrow of our bones.
Bones provide support for muscles that allow movement—muscles attach to bones via tendons, and we are able to move all of our joints because of the connections between our muscles and our bones.	

Table 9.1
Functions of Bone in the Human Body

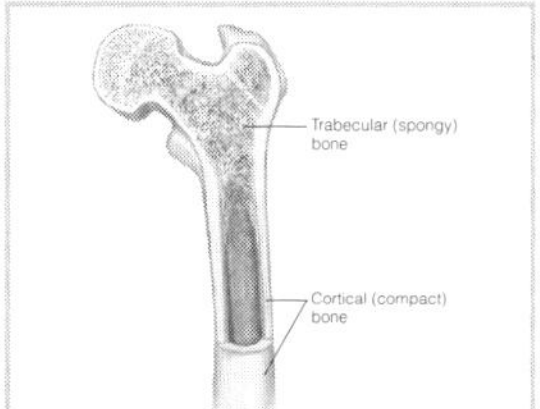

Figure 9.1
The structure of bone.

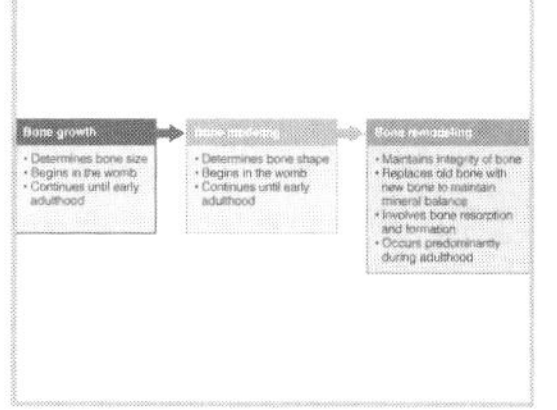

Figure 9.2
Bone growth, bone modeling, and bone remodeling.

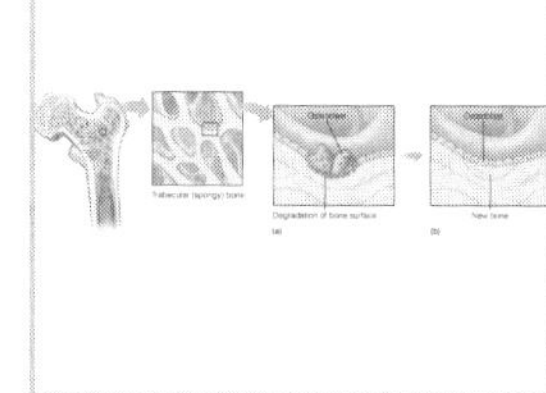

Figure 9.3
Bone remodeling involves resorption and formation.

Activity:

To demonstrate the necessity of mineral deposition in bone, obtain 2 chicken or turkey bones (the drumsticks are the best choice). Soak one of the bones in vinegar for about one week. If the bone is still hard, replace the vinegar and soak a few more days. Check to see when the bone becomes soft. Bring both bones to class and show students the difference between the two bones. Explain that the acetic acid in the vinegar dissolved the mineral salts in the soaked bone, leaving only the bone matrix.

II. How Do We Assess Bone Health? (p. 365)

Key Terms: dual energy x-ray absorptiometry (DXA or DEXA), T-score

Instructor Tools: Chapter 9 PPT slides, Chapter 9 PRS Clicker Questions slide 2, TA 205

Image:

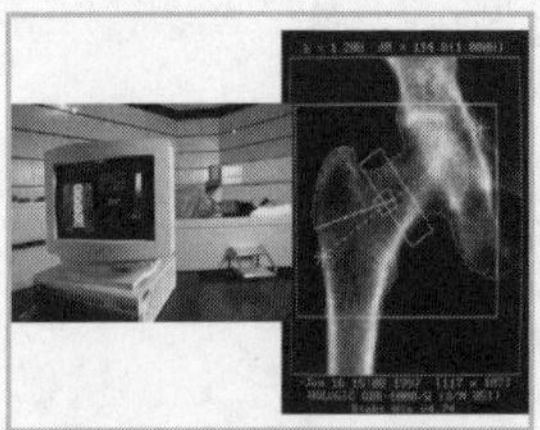

Figure 9.4
Dual energy x-ray absorptiometry.

III. A Profile of Nutrients That Maintain Bone Health (p. 366)

a. Calcium
b. Shopper's Guide: Good Food Sources of Calcium
c. Vitamin D
d. Shopper's Guide: Good Food Sources of Vitamin D
e. Vitamin K
f. Phosphorus
g. Magnesium
h. Fluoride

Key Terms: parathyroid hormone (PTH), calcitonin, bioavailability, hypercalcemia, hypocalcemia, calcitriol, ergocalciferol, cholecalciferol, rickets, osteomalacia, phylloquinone, menaquinone, coenzyme, cofactor, hypermagnesemia, hypomagnesemia, fluorohydroxyapatite, fluorosis

Instructor Tools: Chapter 9 PPT slides, Chapter 9 PRS Clicker Questions slides 3–5, TAs 206–217, 221–224

Animation: *Activation of Vitamin D*

Images:

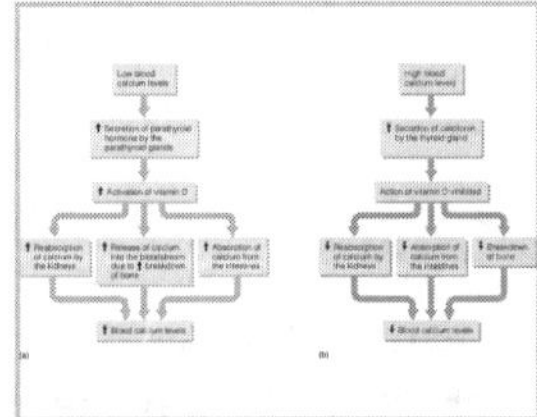

Figure 9.5
Regulation of blood calcium levels by various organs and hormones.

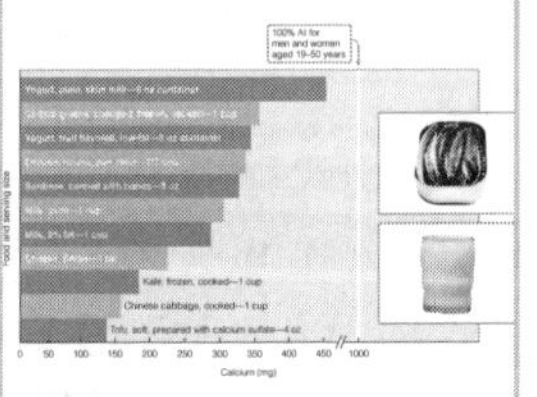

Figure 9.6
Common food sources of calcium.

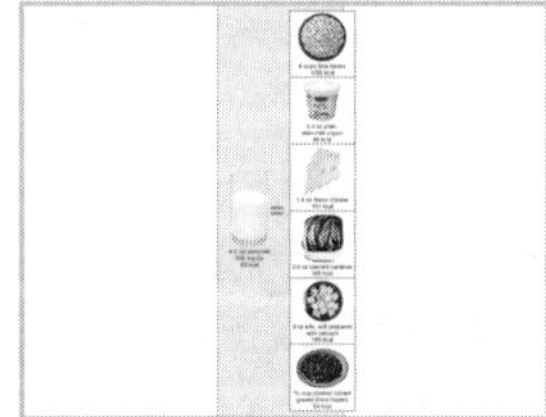

Figure 9.7
Serving sizes and energy content of various foods that contain the same amount of calcium as an 8-fluid ounce glass of skim milk.

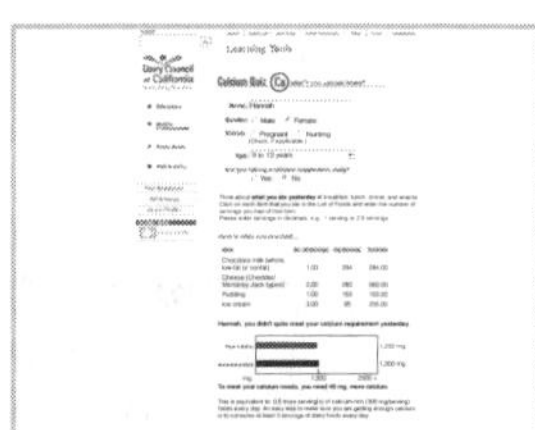

Figure 9.8
Calcium intake quiz.

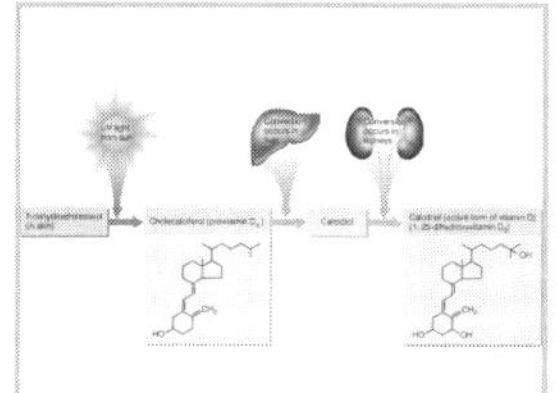

Figure 9.9
Converting sunlight into vitamin D in our skin.

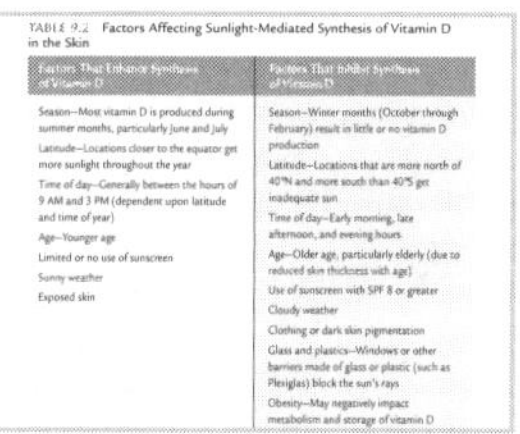

TABLE 9.2 Factors Affecting Sunlight-Mediated Synthesis of Vitamin D in the Skin

Factors That Enhance Synthesis of Vitamin D	Factors That Inhibit Synthesis of Vitamin D
Season—Most vitamin D is produced during summer months, particularly June and July	Season—Winter months (October through February) result in little or no vitamin D production
Latitude—Locations closer to the equator get more sunlight throughout the year	Latitude—Locations that are more north of 40°N and more south than 40°S get inadequate sun
Time of day—Generally between the hours of 9 AM and 3 PM (dependent upon latitude and time of year)	Time of day—Early morning, late afternoon, and evening hours
Age—Younger age	Age—Older age, particularly elderly (due to reduced skin thickness with age)
Limited or no use of sunscreen	Use of sunscreen with SPF 8 or greater
Sunny weather	Cloudy weather
Exposed skin	Clothing or dark skin pigmentation
	Glass and plastics—Windows or other barriers made of glass or plastic (such as Plexiglas) block the sun's rays
	Obesity—May negatively impact metabolism and storage of vitamin D

Table 9.2
Factors Affecting Sunlight-Mediated Synthesis of Vitamin D in the Skin

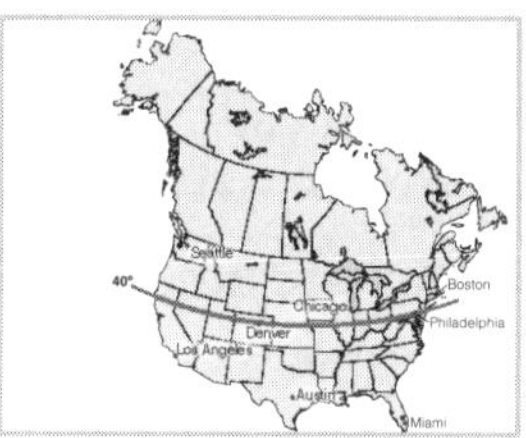

Figure 9.10
The geographical location of 40° latitude in the United States.

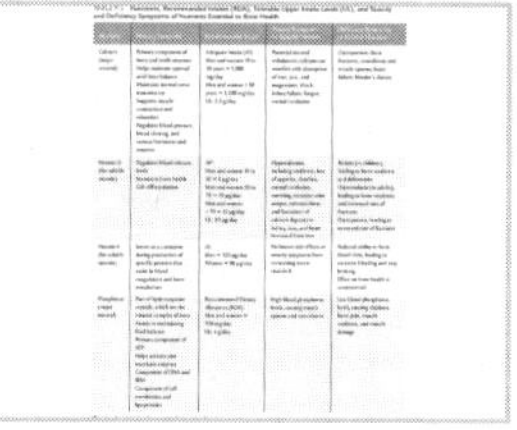

Table 9.3
Recommended Intakes and Toxicity and Deficiency Symptoms of Nutrients Essential to Bone Health

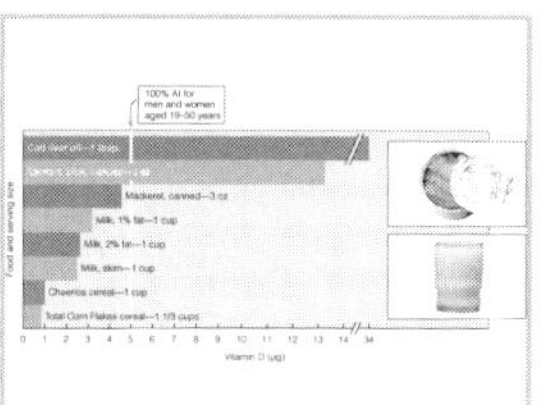

Figure 9.11
Common food sources of vitamin D.

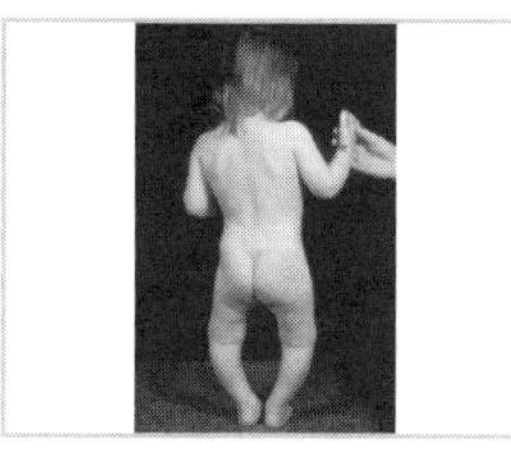

Figure 9.12
Rickets.

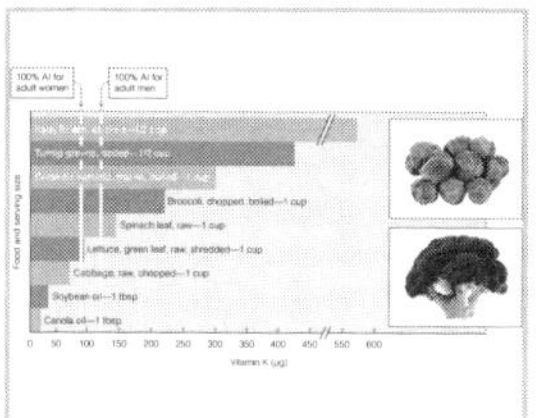

Figure 9.13
Common food sources of vitamin K.

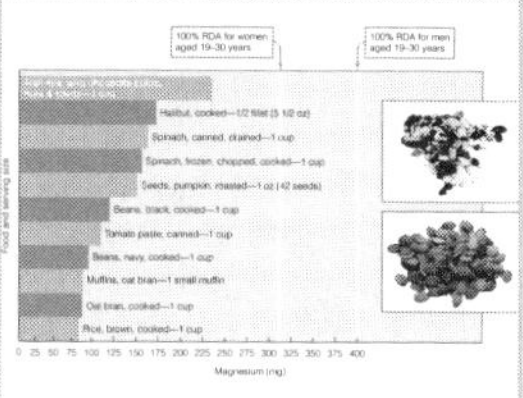

Figure 9.14
Common food sources of magnesium.

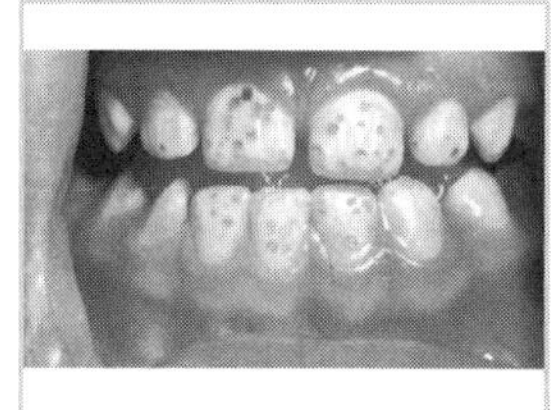

Figure 9.15
Fluorosis, staining and pitting of the teeth.

Activities:

1. Have students work in groups to devise a one-day meal plan with 1,200 mg of calcium. Have them devise a second plan that does not include drinking milk. Discuss with the class which foods provided most of the calcium in each plan.
2. Although most students know dairy is a good source of calcium, they are less likely to be aware of good sources of some of the other nutrients discussed in this chapter. Have students work in small groups to find 3 to 5 significant sources of each of the following:
   - Vitamin D
   - Vitamin K
   - Phosphorus
   - Magnesium

   Ask students to use food composition tables to find the amount of each of these nutrients in the foods they choose. You may also ask them to include the amounts of these foods that would need to be consumed to reach the DRI.

3. To help students learn the nutrients discussed in this chapter, their functions, and their food sources, start by asking a student to name one nutrient. Then ask the next student to add a piece of information about that nutrient. Continue until you get four or five items of information about that nutrient. The next student names another nutrient. Repeat in this manner until all nutrients covered in this chapter have been reviewed.

IV. Osteoporosis Is a Disorder Resulting from Poor Bone Health (p. 388)

a. The Impact of Aging on Osteoporosis Risk

b. Gender and Genetics Affect Osteoporosis Risk

c. Smoking and Poor Nutrition Increase Osteoporosis Risk

d. The Impact of Physical Activity on Osteoporosis Risk

e. Treatments for Osteoporosis

Key Terms: osteoporosis, female athlete triad, antiresorptive

Instructor Tools: Chapter 9 PPT slides, Chapter 9 PRS Clicker Questions slide 6, TAs 218–219, 225

Images:

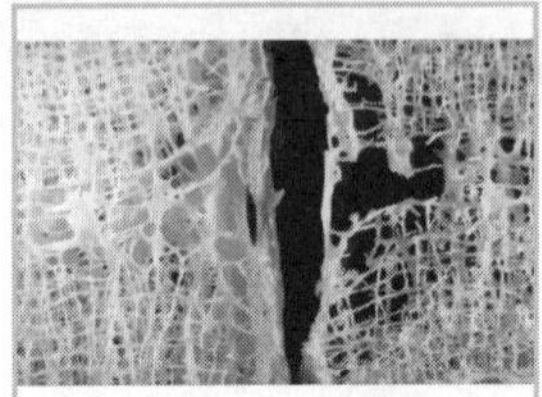

Figure 9.16
Osteoporesis (right) vs. healthy bone (left).

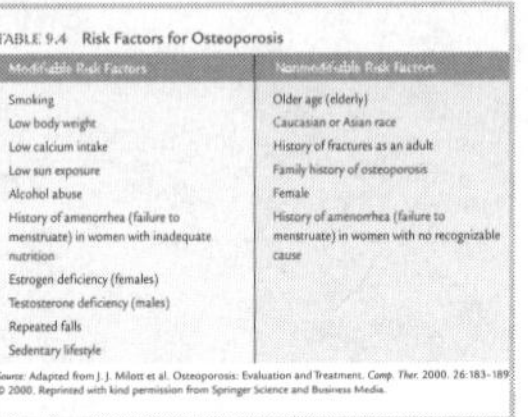

TABLE 9.4 Risk Factors for Osteoporosis

Modifiable Risk Factors	Nonmodifiable Risk Factors
Smoking	Older age (elderly)
Low body weight	Caucasian or Asian race
Low calcium intake	History of fractures as an adult
Low sun exposure	Family history of osteoporosis
Alcohol abuse	Female
History of amenorrhea (failure to menstruate) in women with inadequate nutrition	History of amenorrhea (failure to menstruate) in women with no recognizable cause
Estrogen deficiency (females)	
Testosterone deficiency (males)	
Repeated falls	
Sedentary lifestyle	

Source: Adapted from J. J. Milott et al. Osteoporosis: Evaluation and Treatment. *Comp. Ther.* 2000. 26:183–189 © 2000. Reprinted with kind permission from Springer Science and Business Media.

Table 9.4
Risk Factors for Osteoporosis

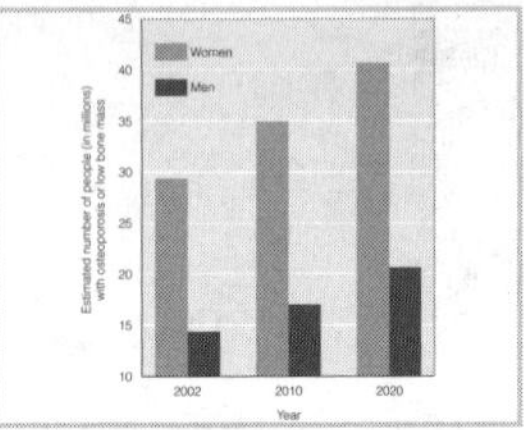

Figure 9.17
The prevalence of osteoporosis and low bone mass.

Activity:

To demonstrate the amount of calcium present in the body at various stages of the life cycle, obtain five clear plastic bags. Using flour to represent calcium, add the following amounts of flour to the bags:

¼ cup flour	represents 27 g calcium	present in the newborn
3½ cup flour	represents 400 g calcium	present in a 10-year-old
7 cups flour	represents 800 g calcium	present in a 15-year-old
11 cups flour	represents 1,200 g calcium	present in an adult
6½ cups flour	represents 750 g calcium	present in osteoporosis

V. Additional Chapter 9 Instructor Tools

MyDietAnalysis Activity: Using the nutritional assessment previously completed, students should note the following:

1. How many grams of calcium do you consume daily?
2. How many micrograms of vitamin D do you consume daily?

3. How many milligrams of magnesium do you consume daily?
4. How does your intake of these nutrients compare to recommendations?
5. What changes can you make in your diet to more closely meet recommendations?

Nutrition Debate Activity: Divide students into small groups of approximately 4 per group. Assign each group an osteoporosis therapy to research. Some options include:

1. estrogen replacement therapy
2. Fosamax (alendronate)
3. Evista (raloxifene)
4. Miacalcin (calcitonin)

Instruct students to pay special attention to relative risks versus demonstrated benefit. Have students present their findings to the class and debate what the best choices might be.

Printed TestBank: Pages 127–139 (TestGen Chapter 9)

MyDietAnalysis Online Assignment: Gustavo: Food, Nutrients, and Risk for Developing Chronic Disease

Quiz Show PowerPoints: Chapter 9

Notes

Nutrients Involved in Energy Metabolism and Blood Health

10

Chapter at a Glance

I. How Do Our Bodies Regulate Energy Metabolism?
II. A Profile of Nutrients Involved in Energy Metabolism
III. What Is the Role of Blood in Maintaining Health?
IV. A Profile of Nutrients That Maintain Healthy Blood

Visual Lecture Outline

I. How Do Our Bodies Regulate Energy Metabolism? (p. 402)

a. Our Bodies Require Vitamins and Minerals to Produce Energy

b. Some Micronutrients Assist with Nutrient Transport and Hormone Production

Key Term: coenzyme

Instructor Tools: Chapter 10 PPT slides, Chapter 10 PRS Clicker Questions slide 1, TAs 226–227

Images:

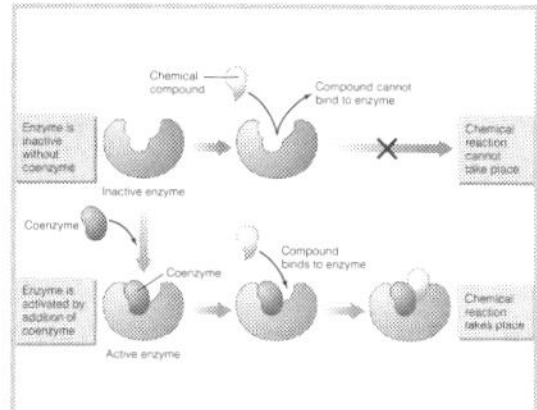

Figure 10.1
Coenzyme activity.

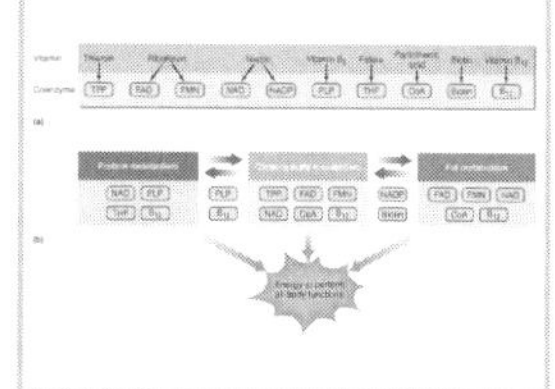

Figure 10.2
B-complex vitamins and coenzymes.

II. A Profile of Nutrients Involved in Energy Metabolism (p. 404)

a. Thiamin (Vitamin B_1)

b. Riboflavin (Vitamin B_2)

c. Niacin

d. Vitamin B_6 (Pyridozine)

e. Folate

f. Vitamin B_{12} (Cobalamin)

g. Pantothenic Acid

h. Biotin

i. Choline

j. Iodine

k. Chromium

l. Manganese

m. Sulfur

Key Terms: beriberi, ariboflavinosis, pellagra, homocysteine, neural tube defects, macrocytic anemia, pernicious anemia, atrophic gastritis, intrinsic factor, acetylcholine, goiter, cretinism

Instructor Tools: Chapter 10 PPT slides, Chapter 10 PRS Clicker Questions slides 2–3, TAs 228–236, 243–246

Animation: *Vitamin B_{12} Absorption*

Images:

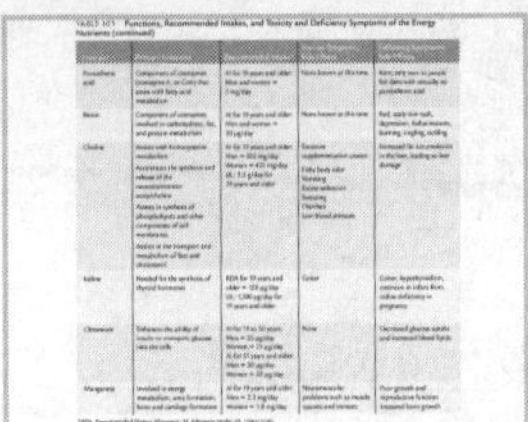

Table 10.1
Energy Nutrients

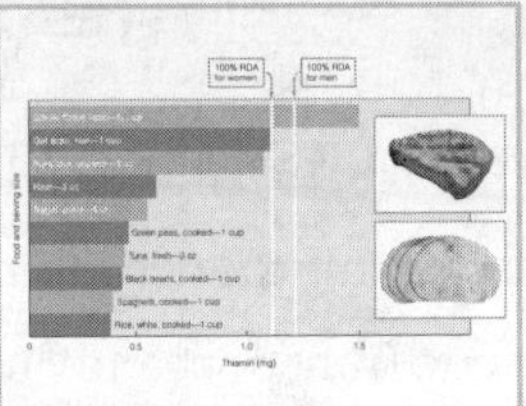

Figure 10.3
Common food sources of thiamin.

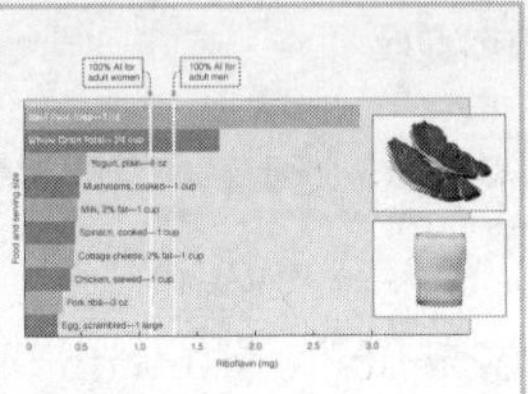

Figure 10.4
Common food sources of riboflavin.

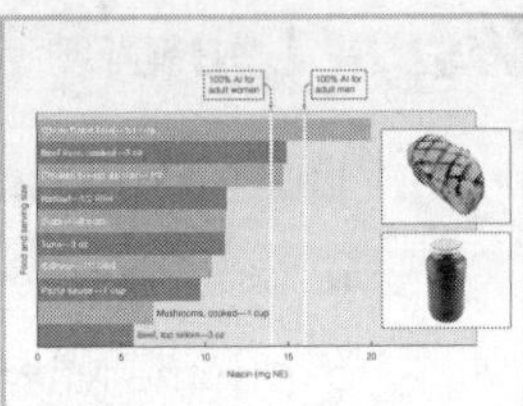

Figure 10.5
Common food sources of niacin.

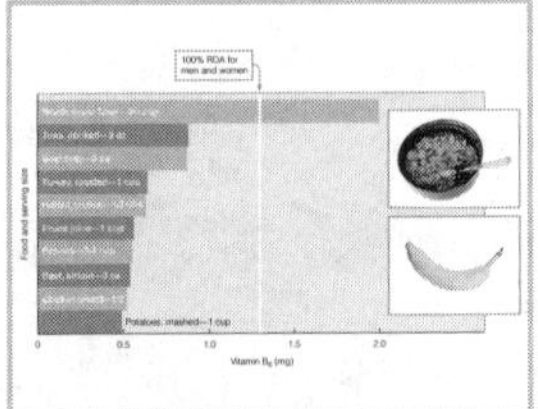

Figure 10.6
Common food sources of vitamin B_6.

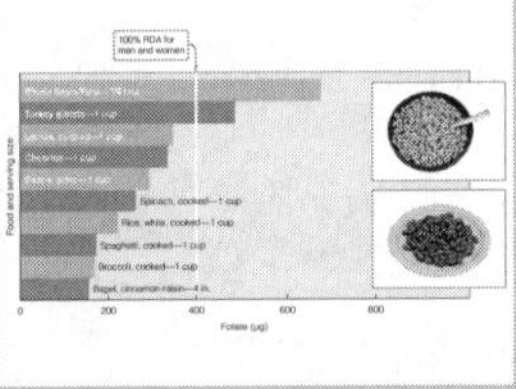

Figure 10.7
Common food sources of folate and folic acid.

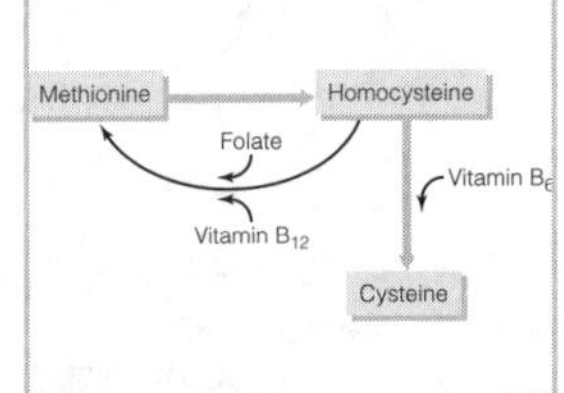

Figure 10.8
The metabolism of methionine to homocysteine.

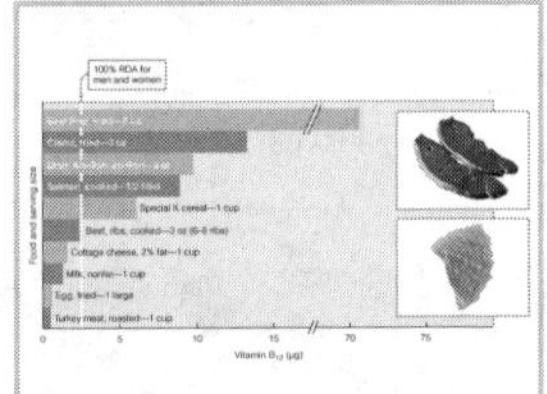

Figure 10.9
Common food sources of vitamin B_{12}.

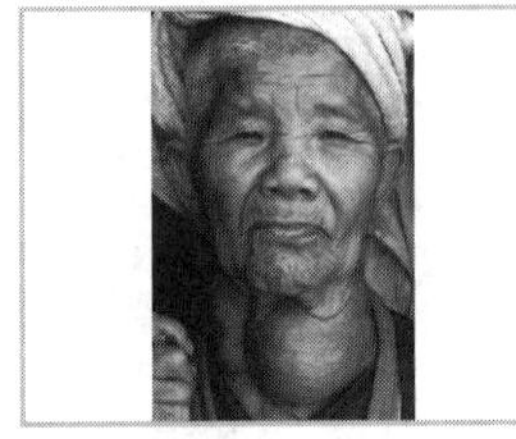

Figure 10.10
Goiter.

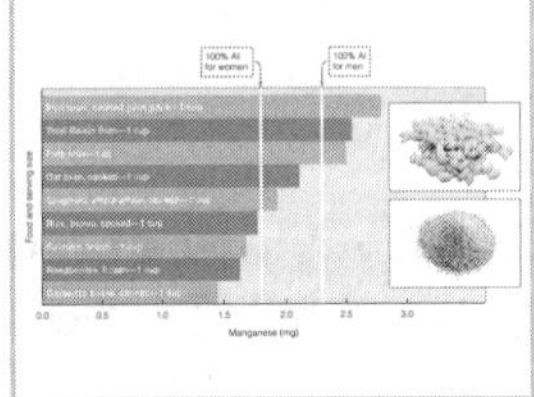

Figure 10.11
Common food sources of manganese.

III. What Is the Role of Blood in Maintaining Health? (p. 421)

Key Terms: erythrocytes, leukocytes, platelets, plasma

Instructor Tools: Chapter 10 PPT slides, TA 237

Image:

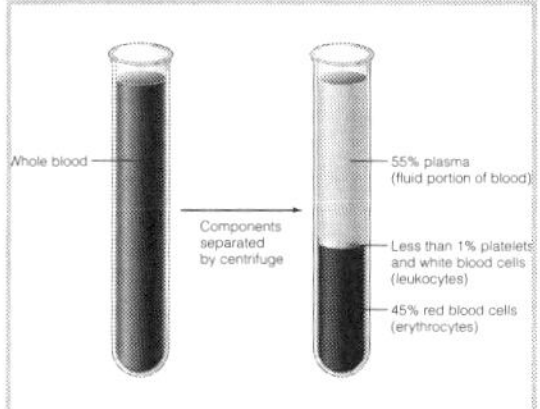

Figure 10.12
Blood has four components.

IV. A Profile of Nutrients That Maintain Healthy Blood (p. 421)

a. Vitamin K

b. Iron

c. Shopper's Guide: Good Food Sources of Iron

d. Zinc

e. Copper

Key Terms: hemoglobin, heme, myoglobin, ferritin, hemosiderin, heme iron, non-heme iron, meat factor, transferrin, iron-deficiency anemia

Instructor Tools: Chapter 10 PPT slides 000–000, Chapter 10 PRS Clicker Questions slides 4–6, TAs 238–242, 247–249

Images:

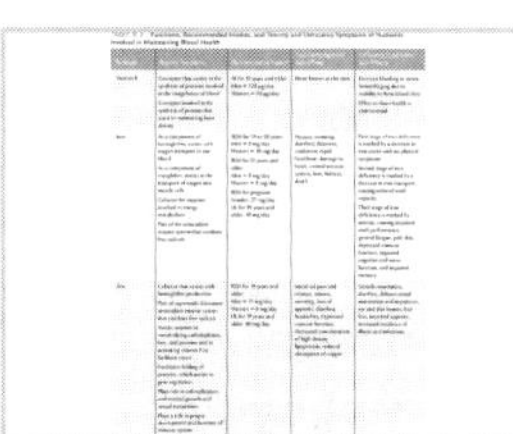

Table 10.2
Nutrient Involved in Maintaining Blood Health

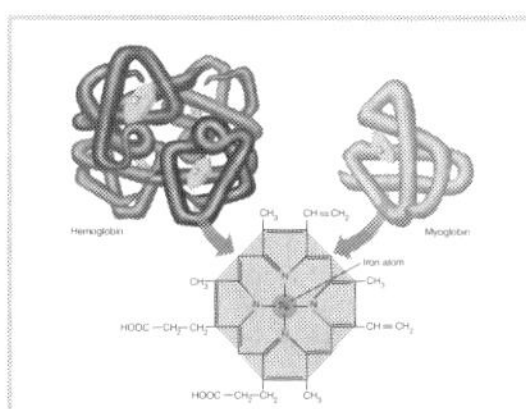

Figure 10.13
Iron is contained in the heme portion of hemoglobin and myoglobin.

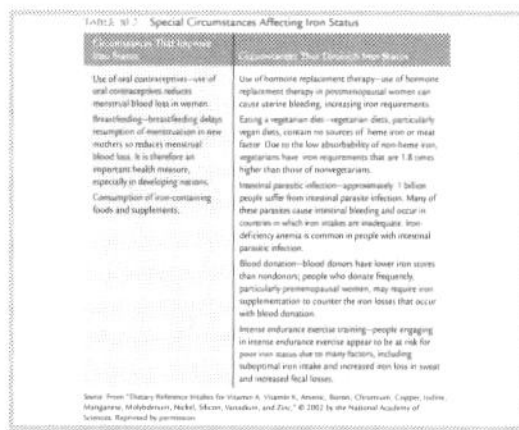

Table 10.3
Special Circumstances Affecting Iron Stores

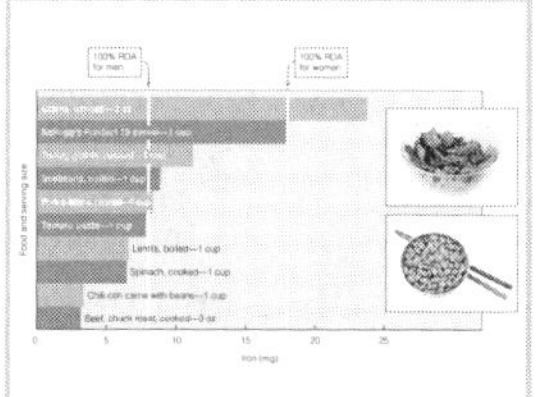

Figure 10.14
Common food sources of iron.

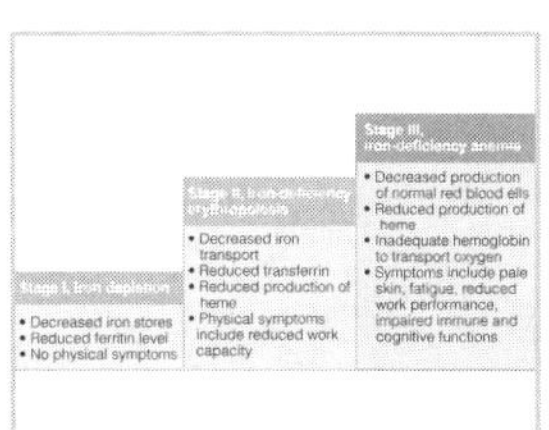

Figure 10.15
Iron deficiency passes through three stages.

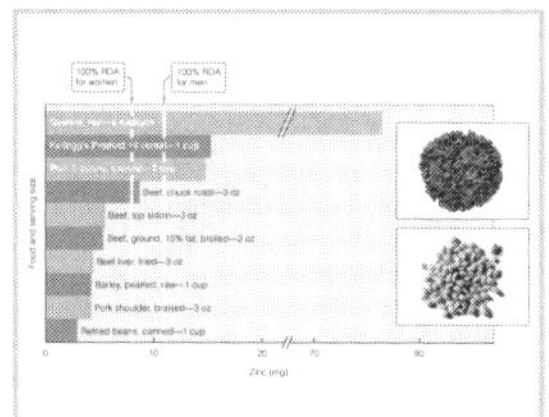

Figure 10.16
Common food sources of zinc.

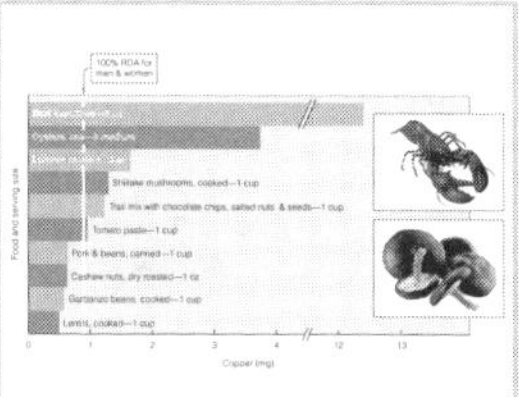

Figure 10.17
Common food sources of copper.

Activities:

1. To help students learn the nutrients discussed in this chapter, their functions, and their food sources, start by asking a student to name one nutrient. Then ask the next student to add a piece of information about that nutrient. Continue until you get four or five items of information about that nutrient. The next student names another nutrient. Repeat in this manner until all nutrients covered in this chapter have been reviewed.
2. Give each student the name of a nutrient or key word covered in the chapter. Ask the students to write a sentence using their assigned word. Collect the sentences and combine them on a worksheet, replacing the key word in each sentence with a blank line. At the end of the worksheet, list all removed key terms alphabetically. Have students complete the worksheet, filling in the blanks with the correct word.
3. Have students find several food products in their home or the grocery store that contain some of the added vitamins and/or minerals covered in this chapter. Then discuss the reasons for adding the nutrients to these products and the potential benefits to consumers.

V. Additional Chapter 10 Instructor Tools

MyDietAnalysis Activity: Using the nutritional assessment previously completed, students should note the following:

a. What is your daily intake of:
   - folate?
   - iron?
   - zinc?

b. How does your intake of these nutrients compare with recommendations?

c. What changes can you make in your diet to more closely meet recommendations?

Nutrition Debate Activity: Ask students to bring in package labels or information obtained from the Internet on various zinc lozenges. Ask them to note the following:

a. What is the cost of the product?

b. What is the suggested dosage of the product?

c. What additional ingredients are present in the product?

Discuss with class members whether they believe these products are worth taking to reduce the length or severity of a cold.

Printed TestBank: Pages 140–153 (TestGen Chapter 10)

Quiz Show PowerPoints: Chapter 10

Achieving and Maintaining a Healthful Body Weight 11

Chapter at a Glance

I. What Is a Healthful Body Weight?
II. How Can You Evaluate Your Body Weight?
III. What Makes Us Gain and Lose Weight?
IV. How Can You Achieve and Maintain a Healthful Body Weight?
V. What Disorders Are Related to Energy Intake?

Visual Lecture Outline

I. What Is a Healthful Body Weight? (p. 442)

Key Terms: underweight, overweight, obesity, morbid obesity

Instructor Tools: Chapter 11 PPT slides, Chapter 11 PRS Clicker Questions slide 1

II. How Can You Evaluate Your Body Weight? (p. 442)

a. Determine Your Body Mass Index (BMI)
b. Measure Your Body Composition
c. Assess Your Fat Distribution Patterns

Key Terms: body mass index (BMI), body composition

Instructor Tools: Chapter 11 PPT slides, TAs 250–255

Images:

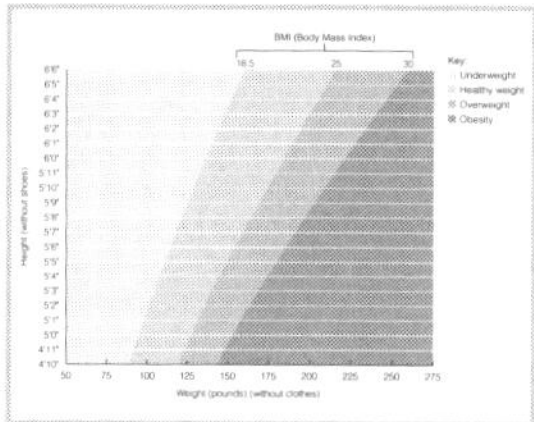

Figure 11.1
BMI graph.

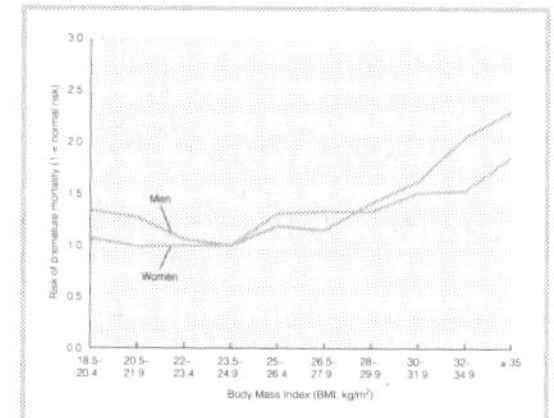

Figure 11.2
BMI vs. increased risk for premature mortality.

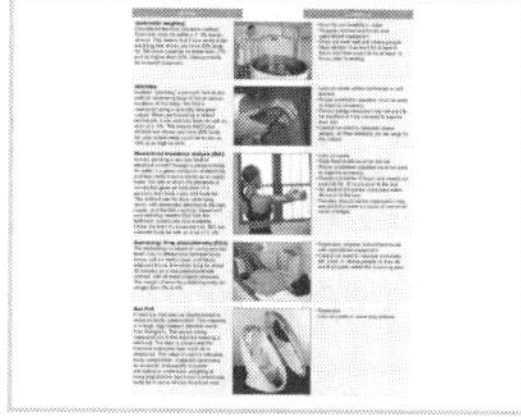

Figure 11.3
Overview of body composition assessment methods.

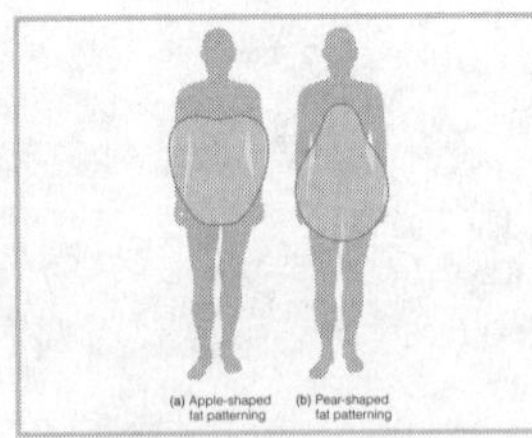

Figure 11.4
Apple- and pear-shaped fat distribution patterns.

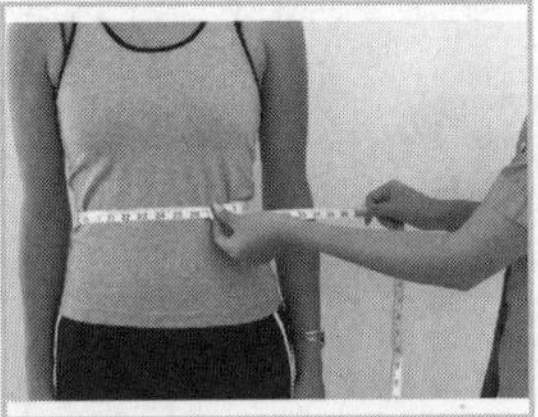

Figure 11.5a
Determining your type of fat patterning.

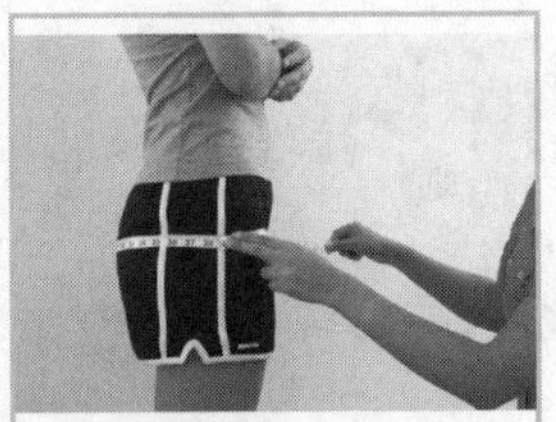

Figure 11.5b
Determininig your type of fat patterning.

Activities:

1. Bring several tape measures to class. Have students measure their waist (at the level of their natural waist) and hip (at the maximal width of the buttocks) circumference. Ask them to:
   a. calculate their waist-to-hip ratio.
   b. compare their waist-to-hip ratio to recommended measurements.
   c. interpret their results.
2. If calipers are available, perform skinfold measurements.
3. Have students calculate their BMI. To do this they must convert their height to meters (divide height in inches by 39.3) and their weight to kilograms (divide weight in pounds by 2.2). They can then calculate BMI using the formula: BMI 5 kg/m^2. Ask students to interpret their BMI with regard to health risks.

III. What Makes Us Gain and Lose Weight? (p. 447)

a. We Gain or Lose Weight When our Energy Intake and Expenditure Are Out of Balance
b. Genetic Factors Affect Body Weight
c. Lifestyle Choices Adopted in Childhood Influence Adult Weight
d. Composition of the Diet Affects Fat Storage
e. Physiologic Factors Influence Body Weight
f. Other Physiologic Factors
g. Psychological and Social Factors Influence Behavior and Body Weight

Key Terms: energy intake, energy expenditure, basal metabolic rate (BMR), thermic effect of food (TEF), energy cost of physical activity, thrifty gene theory, set-point theory, leptin, ghrelin, peptide YY

Instructor Tools: Chapter 11 PPT slides, Chapter 11 PRS Clicker Questions slides 2–4, TAs 256–259, 263–264

Images:

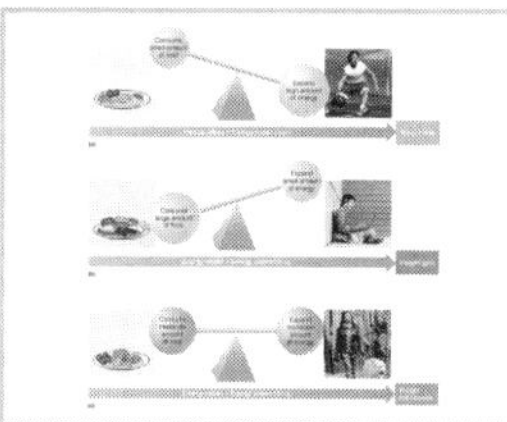

Figure 11.6
Energy balance.

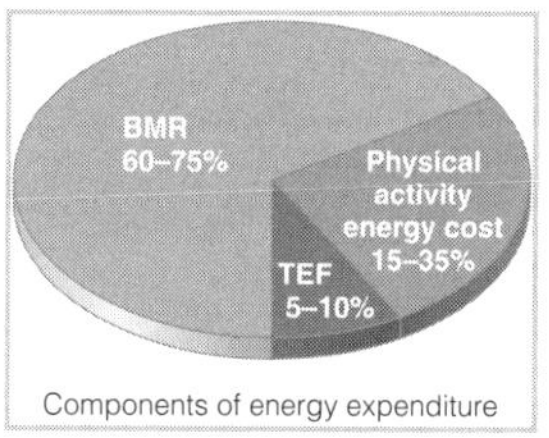

Components of energy expenditure

Figure 11.7
Components of energy expenditure.

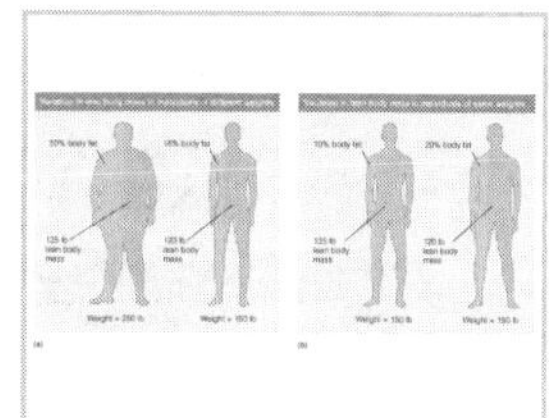

Figure 11.8
Lean body mass variations with different body weights and body fat levels.

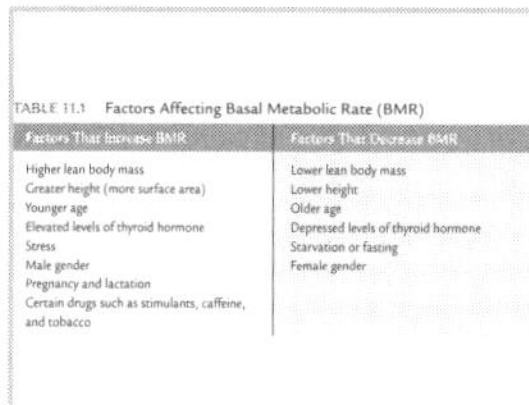

TABLE 11.1 Factors Affecting Basal Metabolic Rate (BMR)

Factors That Increase BMR	Factors That Decrease BMR
Higher lean body mass	Lower lean body mass
Greater height (more surface area)	Lower height
Younger age	Older age
Elevated levels of thyroid hormone	Depressed levels of thyroid hormone
Stress	Starvation or fasting
Male gender	Female gender
Pregnancy and lactation	
Certain drugs such as stimulants, caffeine, and tobacco	

Table 11.1
Factors Affecting Basal Metabolic Rate (BMR)

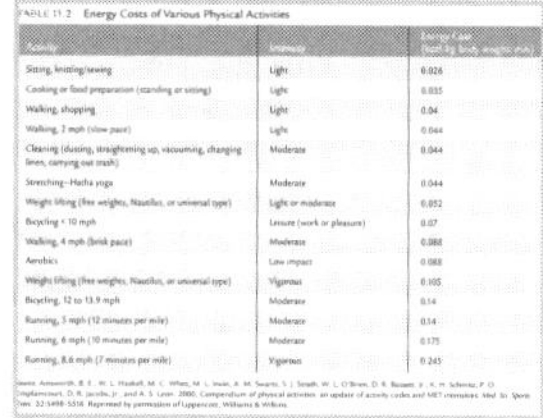

TABLE 11.2 Energy Costs of Various Physical Activities

Activity	Intensity	Energy Cost [illegible]
Sitting, knitting/sewing	Light	0.026
Cooking or food preparation (standing or sitting)	Light	0.035
Walking, shopping	Light	0.04
Walking, 2 mph (slow pace)	Light	0.044
Cleaning (dusting, straightening up, vacuuming, changing linen, carrying out trash)	Moderate	0.044
Stretching–Hatha yoga	Moderate	0.044
Weight lifting (free weights, Nautilus, or universal type)	Light or moderate	0.052
Bicycling < 10 mph	Leisure (work or pleasure)	0.07
Walking, 4 mph (brisk pace)	Moderate	0.088
Aerobics	Low impact	0.088
Weight lifting (free weights, Nautilus, or universal type)	Vigorous	0.105
Bicycling, 12 to 13.9 mph	Moderate	0.14
Running, 5 mph (12 minutes per mile)	Moderate	0.14
Running, 6 mph (10 minutes per mile)	Moderate	0.175
Running, 8.6 mph (7 minutes per mile)	Vigorous	0.245

Table 11.2
Energy Costs of Various Physical Activities

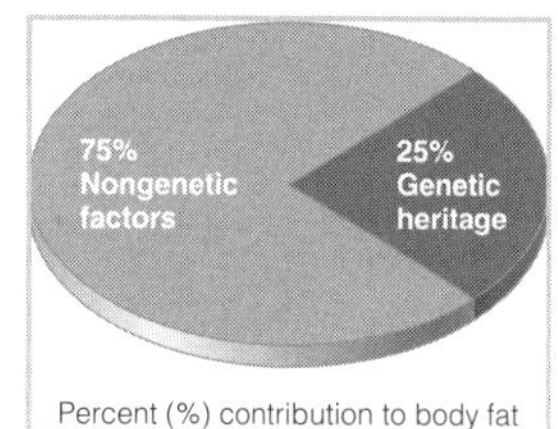

Percent (%) contribution to body fat

Figure 11.9
Genetic and non-genetic contributions to body fat.

IV. How Can You Achieve and Maintain a Healthful Body Weight? (p. 459)

a. If You Decide to Follow a Popular Diet Plan, Choose One Based on the Three Strategies
b. If You Decide to Design Your Own Diet Plan, Include the Three Strategies

abc NEWS Lecture Launcher Video:

Crash Diet

abc NEWS Discussion Questions:

1. Discuss criteria you could use to differentiate a crash diet from a healthful weight loss diet.
2. Although crash diets may result in dramatic weight loss, this weight loss is not necessarily a result of losing only body fat. Discuss the possible reasons for this and implications for maintaining this weight for the long term.
3. What are some potential challenges a dieter would face when following a crash diet like the one described in the "*Crash Diet*" video?

Instructor Tools: Chapter 11 PPT slides, Chapter 11 PRS Clicker Questions slide 5, TAs 260, 265

Images:

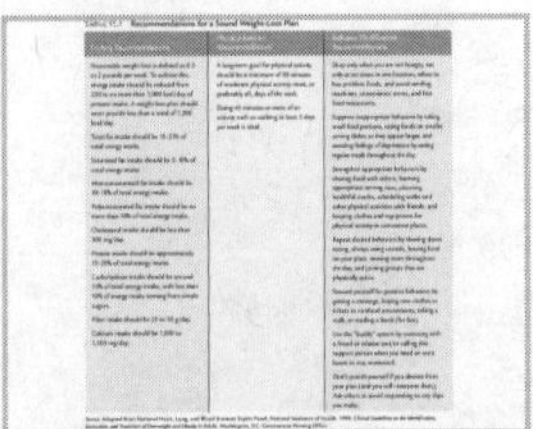

Table 11.3
Recommendations for a Sound Weight-Loss Plan

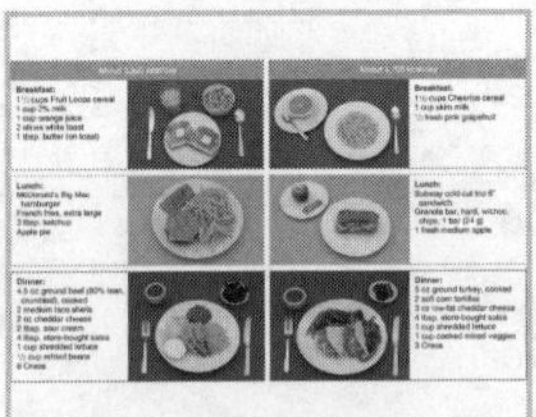

Figure 11.10
The energy density of two sets of meals.

Activity:

Have students work in groups to obtain a copy of a currently popular weight-loss diet and evaluate it. The guidelines described on p. 460–461 can be used to help students recognize fad diets.

V. What Disorders Are Related to Energy Intake? (p. 468)

a. Underweight

b. Overweight

c. Obesity and Morbid Obesity

abc NEWS **Lecture Launcher Video:**

Gastric Bypass Surgery

abc NEWS **Video Discussion Questions:**

1. What are potential long term problems that can occur in children after gastric bypass surgery?
2. What are potential risks facing obese children?
3. Do you think the benefits of gastric bypass surgery outweigh the risks in children? Why or why not?

Instructor Tools: Chapter 11 PPT slides 000–000, Chapter 11 PRS Clicker Questions slides 6–7, TAs 261–262

Animation: *Obesity Rates*

Images:

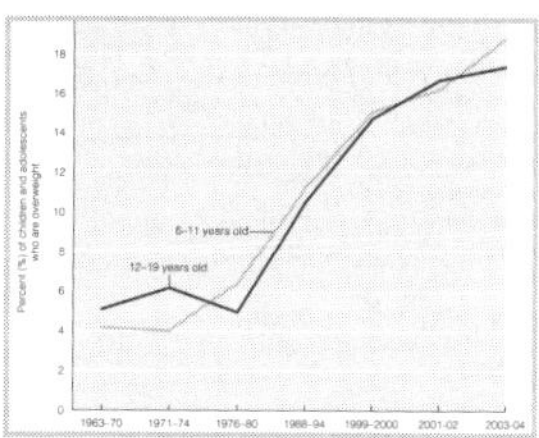

Figure 11.11
Increases in childhood and adolescent overweight from 1963 to 2004.

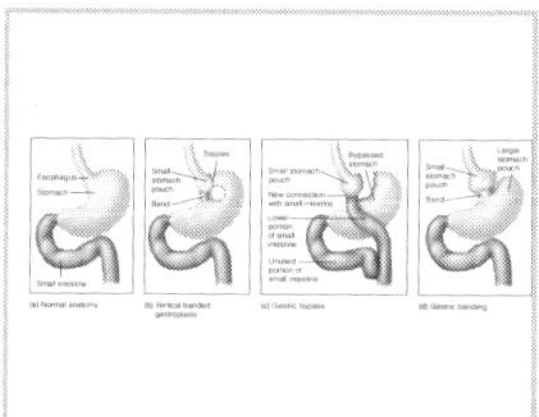

Figure 11.12
Various forms of surgery alter the normal anatomy of the GI tract.

VI. Additional Chapter 11 Instructor Tools

MyDietAnalysis Activity: Using the nutritional assessment previously completed, students should note the following:

a. How many calories do you consume daily?

b. How does this caloric intake compare to recommendations?

c. What three foods that you consume contain the highest number of calories? How many calories are in each food?

d. What changes can you make in your diet to more closely meet caloric recommendations?

Nutrition Debate Activity: Ask students to keep a journal for 1 to 3 days with observations in their daily life that may contribute to weight gain and/or weight loss. In class, students can share their observations and discuss possible changes that can help maintain a healthy weight.

Some examples of conditions to note might include:

a. presence or absence of sidewalks

b. presence or absence of bicycle lanes

c. parks or other open space in their area

d. cost of foods in the grocery store

e. presence or absence of fast food restaurants

f. availability of healthy food at their school or workplace

Printed TestBank: Pages 154–166 (TestGen Chapter 11)

MyDietAnalysis Online Assignment: Nadia and Laurie: Similar Needs and Different Intakes

Quiz Show PowerPoints: Chapter 11

Notes

Nutrition and Physical Activity: Keys to Good Health

12

Chapter at a Glance

I. Why Engage in Physical Activity?
II. What Is a Sound Fitness Program?
III. What Fuels Our Activities?
IV. What Kind of Diet Supports Physical Activity?
V. Are Ergogenic Aids Necessary for Active People?

Visual Lecture Outline

I. Why Engage in Physical Activity? (p. 484)

Key Terms: physical activity, leisure-time physical activity, exercise, physical fitness, cardiorespiratory fitness, musculoskeletal fitness, muscular strength, muscular endurance, flexibility, body composition

Instructor Tools: Chapter 12 PPT slides, TAs 266, 277

Images:

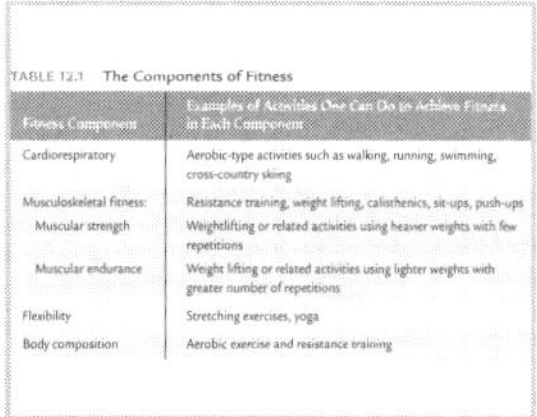

TABLE 12.1 The Components of Fitness

Fitness Component	Examples of Activities One Can Do to Achieve Fitness in Each Component
Cardiorespiratory	Aerobic-type activities such as walking, running, swimming, cross-country skiing
Musculoskeletal fitness:	Resistance training, weight lifting, calisthenics, sit-ups, push-ups
Muscular strength	Weightlifting or related activities using heavier weights with few repetitions
Muscular endurance	Weight lifting or related activities using lighter weights with greater number of repetitions
Flexibility	Stretching exercises, yoga
Body composition	Aerobic exercise and resistance training

Table 12.1
The Components of Fitness

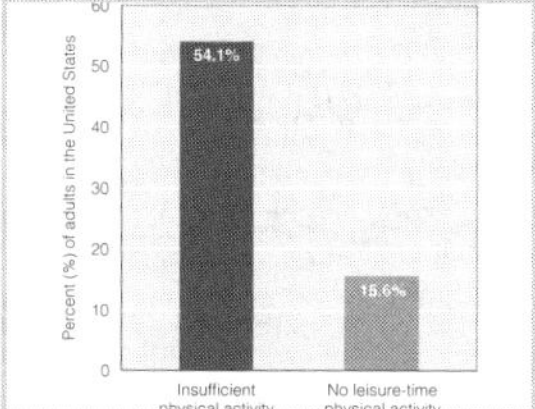

Figure 12.1
Rates of physical inactivity in the United States.

II. What Is a Sound Fitness Program? (p. 486)

a. A Sound Fitness Program Meets Your Personal Goals
b. A Sound Fitness Program Is Fun and Includes Variety and Consistency
c. A Sound Fitness Program Appropriately Overloads the Body
d. A Sound Fitness Plan Includes a Warm-Up and a Cool-Down Period

Key Terms: Physical Activity Pyramid, resistance training, overload principle, FIT principle, frequency, intensity, low-intensity activities, moderate-intensity activities, vigorous-intensity activities, maximal heart rate, time of activity, warm-up, cool-down

Instructor Tools: Chapter 12 PPT slides, Chapter 12 PRS Clicker Questions slide 1, TAs 267–269, 278

Images:

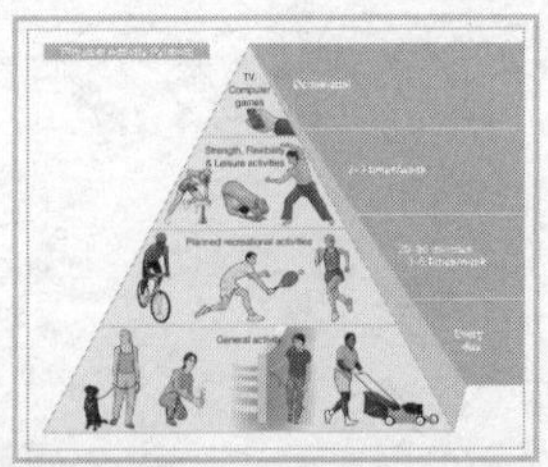
Figure 12.2
Physical Activity Pyramid.

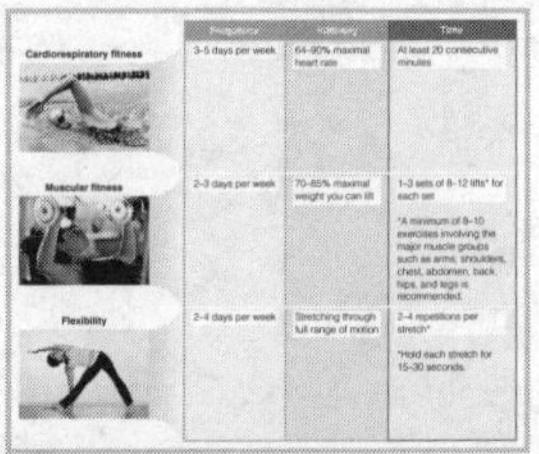
Figure 12.3
The FIT principle.

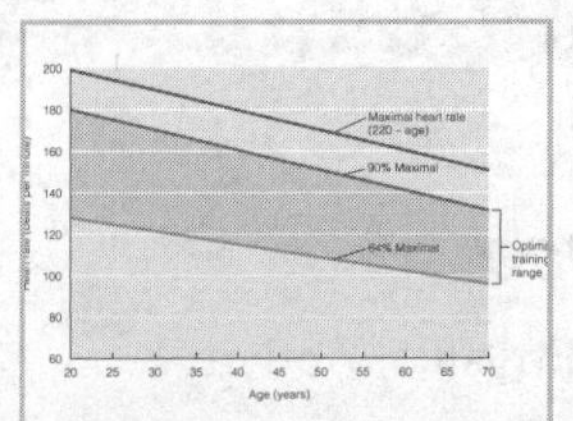
Figure 12.4
This heart rate training chart can be used to estimate your aerobic exercise intensity.

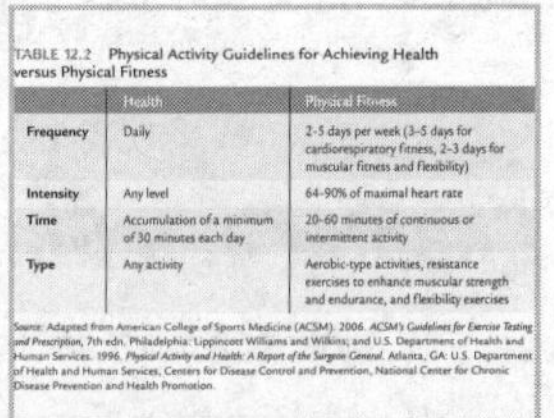
TABLE 12.2 Physical Activity Guidelines for Achieving Health versus Physical Fitness

	Health	Physical Fitness
Frequency	Daily	2-5 days per week (3–5 days for cardiorespiratory fitness, 2–3 days for muscular fitness and flexibility)
Intensity	Any level	64-90% of maximal heart rate
Time	Accumulation of a minimum of 30 minutes each day	20-60 minutes of continuous or intermittent activity
Type	Any activity	Aerobic-type activities, resistance exercises to enhance muscular strength and endurance, and flexibility exercises

Source: Adapted from American College of Sports Medicine (ACSM). 2006. *ACSM's Guidelines for Exercise Testing and Prescription*, 7th edn. Philadelphia: Lippincott Williams and Wilkins; and U.S. Department of Health and Human Services. 1996. *Physical Activity and Health: A Report of the Surgeon General*. Atlanta, GA: U.S. Department of Health and Human Services, Centers for Disease Control and Prevention, National Center for Chronic Disease Prevention and Health Promotion.

Table 12.2
Physical Activity Guidelines for Achieving Health versus Physical Fitness

Activity:

Instruct students to measure their resting pulse. Have students classify themselves as sedentary, moderately active, or very active. Record pulse rates for students in each category. It is a good idea to discuss with the class the difference between busy and active before students classify themselves.

III. What Fuels Our Activities? (p. 493)

a. The ATP-CP Energy System Uses Creatine Phosphate to Regenerate ATP
b. The Breakdown of Carbohydrates Provides Energy for Brief and Long-Term Exercise
c. Aerobic Breakdown of Fats Supports Exercise of Low Intensity and Long Duration
d. Amino Acids Are Not Major Sources of Fuel During Exercise

Key Terms: adenosine triphosphate (ATP), creatine phosphate (CP), anaerobic, glycolysis, pyruvic acid, lactic acid

Instructor Tools: Chapter 12 PPT slides, Chapter 12 PRS Clicker Questions slides 2–3, TAs 270–274

Animation: *Energy Currency, Glycolysis, Cori Cycle*

Images:

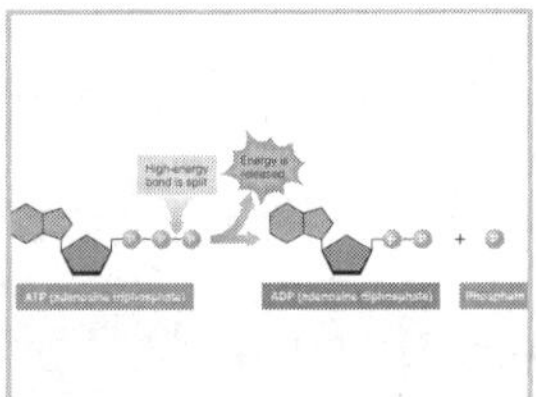
Figure 12.5
Structure of adenosine triphosphate (ATP).

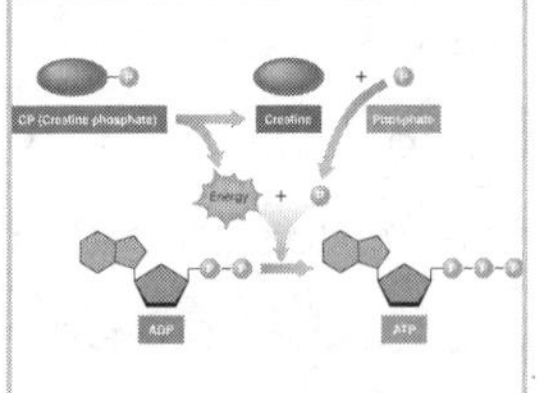
Figure 12.6
Regeneration of ATP.

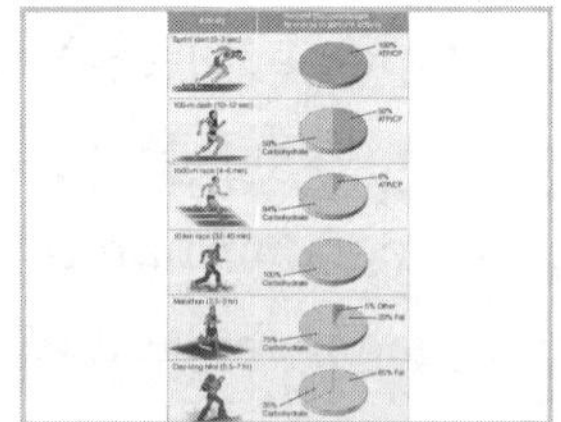
Figure 12.7
Relative contributions of ATP-CP, carbohydrate, and fat to activities of various durations and intensities.

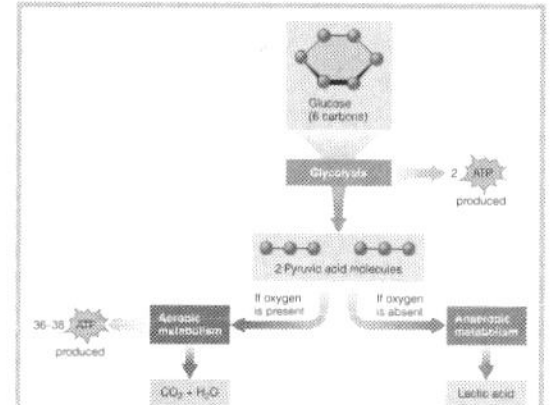

Figure 12.8
The process of glycolysis yields two molecules of pyruvic acid and two ATP molecules.

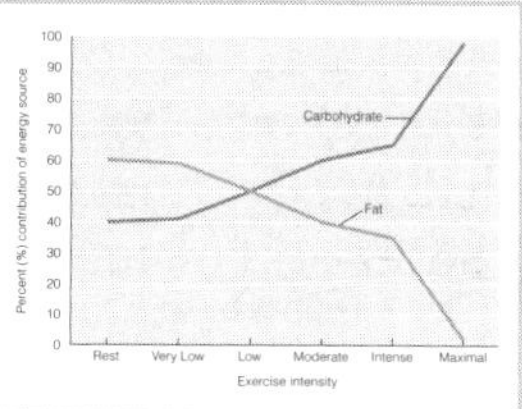

Figure 12.9
For most daily activities, including exercise, we use a mixture of carbohydrate and fat for energy.

IV. What Kind of Diet Supports Physical Activity? (p. 499)

a. Vigorous Exercise Increases Energy Needs

b. Carbohydrate Needs Increase for Many Active People

c. Moderate Fat Consumption Is Enough to Support Most Activities

d. Active People Need More Protein Than Do Inactive People, but Many Already Eat Enough

e. Regular Exercise Increases Our Need for Fluids

f. Inadequate Intakes of Some Vitamins and Minerals Can Diminish Health and Performance

Instructor Tools: Chapter 12 PPT slides, Chapter 12 PRS Clicker Questions slide 4, TAs 275–276, 279–287

Images:

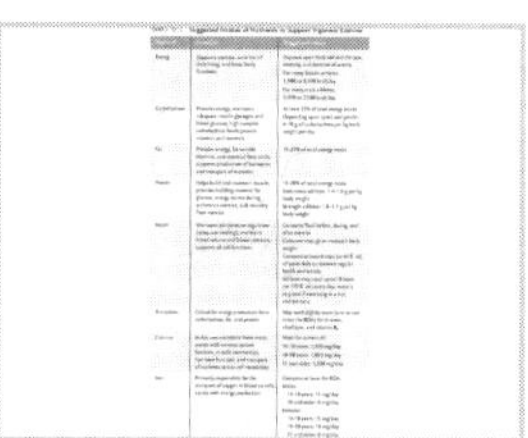

Table 12.3
Suggested Intakes of Nutrients to Support Vigorous Exercise

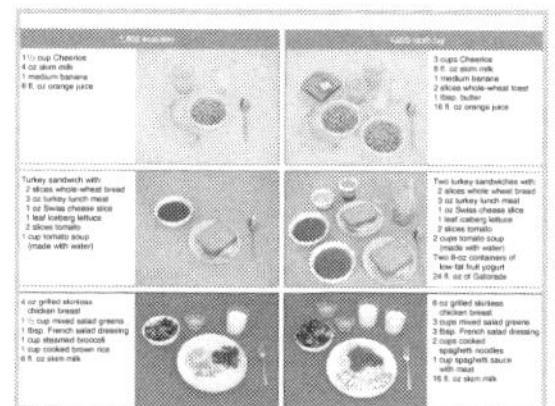

Figure 12.10
High-carbohydrate meals at two kcal levels.

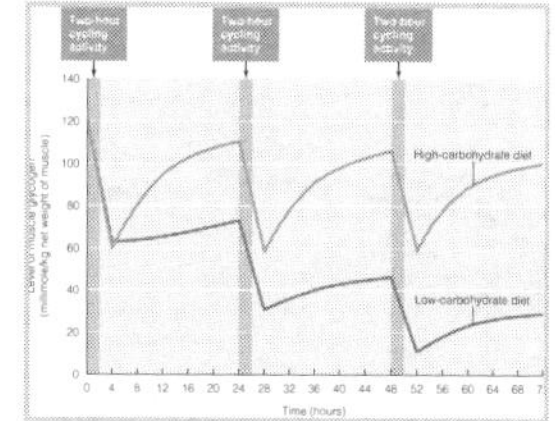

Figure 12.11
The effects of a low carbohydrate diet on muscle glycogen stores.

Table 12.4
Carbohydrate and Total Energy in Various Foods and Sport Bars

TABLE 12.5 Recommended Carbohydrate Loading Procedure for Endurance Athletes

Days Prior to Event	Exercise Duration (minutes)	Carbohydrate Content of Diet (grams per kilogram of body weight)
6	90	5
5	40	5
4	40	5
3	20	10
2	20	10
1	None (rest day)	10
Day of Race	Competition	Precompetition food and fluid

Source: Adapted from Coleman, E. 2006. Carbohydrate and exercise. In: Dunford, M., edn. Sports Nutrition, 4th edn. Chicago, IL: The American Dietetic Association. Used with permission.

Table 12.5
Recommended Carbohydrate Loading Procedure for Endurance Athletes

TABLE 12.6 Estimated Protein Requirements for Athletes

Group	Protein Requirements (grams per kilogram body weight)
Competitive male and female athletes	1.4–1.6
Moderate-intensity endurance athletes	1.2
Recreational endurance athletes	0.8–1.0
Football, power sports players	1.4–1.7
Resistance athletes, weight lifters (early training)	1.5–1.7
Resistance athletes, weight lifters (steady-state training)	1.0–1.2

Source: Tarnopolsky, M. 2006. Protein and amino acid needs for training and bulking up. In: Burke, L. and Deakin, V., eds. *Clinical Sports Nutrition*, 3rd edn. Sydney, Australia: McGraw-Hill, p. 109.

Table 12.6
Estimated Protein Requirements for Athletes

TABLE 12.7 Signs of Dehydration During Heavy Exercise

Decreases In:	Increases In:
Exercise performance	Heart rate at a given exercise intensity
Urine output (and urine is dark yellow or brown in color)	Level of perceived exertion during exercise
Appetite	Fatigue and weakness
Ability to mentally concentrate	Headache and dizziness

Table 12.7
Signs of Dehydration During Heavy Exercise

Table 12.8
Guidelines for Fluid Replacement

Activity:

Have students take a poll of their peers with questions about their exercise habits. Ask students to note age and gender for each person polled. In class, make bar graphs for each age group and sex. Examples of questions that can be addressed include:

a. What type of exercise(s) do you do?

b. How many minutes per day is each exercise done?

V. Are Ergogenic Aids Necessary for Active People? (p. 468)

a. Anabolic Products Are Touted as Muscle and Strength Enhancers

b. Some Products Are Said to Optimize Fuel Use During Exercise

Instructor Tools: Chapter 12 PPT slides, Chapter 12 PRS Clicker Questions slide 5

VI. Additional Chapter 12 Instructor Tools

MyDietAnalysis Activities:

1. Have students use the "Activity Tracker" in the MyDietAnalysis software to keep track of their exercise activity for one week. Have them submit an "Activity Summary Report" to the instructor. Discuss in class the calorie expenditures associated with various activities.
2. Using the nutritional assessment previously completed, students should compare their nutrient intake with "Suggested Intakes of Nutrients to Support Vigorous Exercise" in Table 12.3 on p. 500. Ask them to indicate what changes they could make in their diet to more closely meet the recommendations to support vigorous exercise.

Nutrition Debate Activity: Have students develop what they would consider an ideal exercise program for themselves. Have them include:

a. exercises that include all components of fitness listed in Table 12.1 on p. 485

b. a realistic schedule

Printed TestBank: Pages 167–181 (TestGen Chapter 12)

Quiz Show PowerPoints: Chapter 12

Disordered Eating

13

Chapter at a Glance

I. Eating Behaviors Occur on a Continuum
II. What Factors Contribute to the Development of Eating Disorders?
III. What Does an Eating Disorder Look Like?
IV. What Does Disordered Eating Look Like?
V. What Is the Female Athlete Triad?
VI. What Therapies Work for People with an Eating Disorder?
VII. How Can We Prevent Eating Disorders and Disordered Eating?

Visual Lecture Outline

I. Eating Behaviors Occur on a Continuum (p. 526)

a. Feelings About Food and Body Image Influence Eating Behaviors

b. Eating Disorders and Disordered Eating Patterns Are Not the Same Thing

Key Terms: body image, eating disorder, disordered eating

Instructor Tools: Chapter 13 PPT slides 000–000, Chapter 13 PRS Clicker Question slide 1, TAs 288–289

Image:

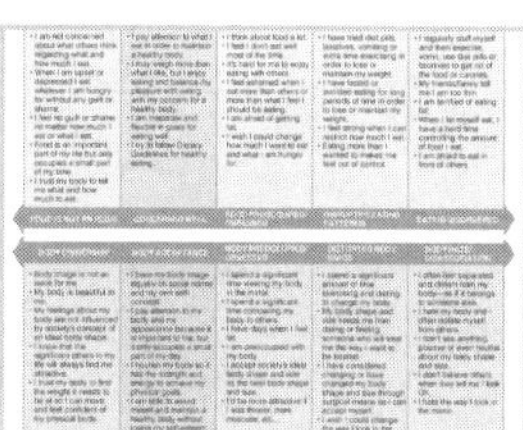

Figure 13.1
The Eating Issues and Body Image Continuum.

II. What Factors Contribute to the Development of Eating Disorders? (p. 528)

a. Family Environment Influences Eating Behavior

b. Sociocultural Values Shape Identity and Self-Esteem

c. Unrealistic Media Images Affect Body Image

d. Certain Personality Traits Are Associated with Eating Disorders

e. Genetic and Biological Factors May Contribute to Eating Disorders

Instructor Tools: Chapter 13 PPT slides, Chapter 13 PRS Clicker Question slide 2, TAs 290–291, 298

Images:

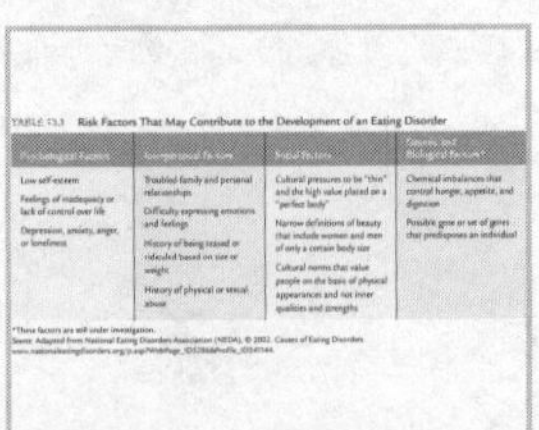

TABLE 13.1 Risk Factors That May Contribute to the Development of an Eating Disorder

[illegible]	[illegible]	[illegible]	Genetic and Biological Factors*
Low self-esteem Feelings of inadequacy or lack of control over life Depression, anxiety, anger, or loneliness	Troubled family and personal relationships Difficulty expressing emotions and feelings History of being teased or ridiculed based on size or weight History of physical or sexual abuse	Cultural pressures to be "thin" and the high value placed on a "perfect body" Narrow definitions of beauty that include women and men of only a certain body size Cultural norms that value people on the basis of physical appearances and not inner qualities and strengths	Chemical imbalances that control hunger, appetite, and digestion Possible gene or set of genes that predisposes an individual

*These factors are still under investigation.
Source: Adapted from National Eating Disorders Association (NEDA), © 2002. Causes of Eating Disorders [illegible]

Table 13.1
Risk Factors that May Contribute to the Development of an Eating Disorder

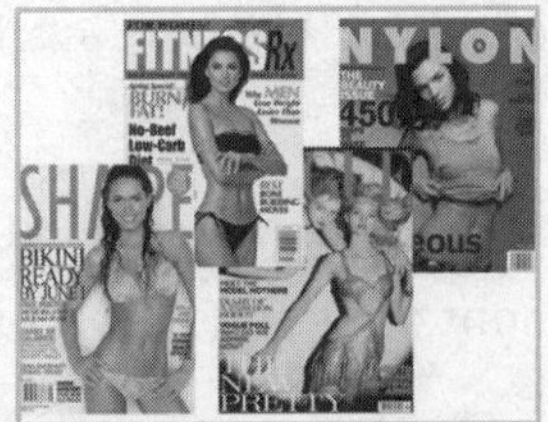

Figure 13.2
Photos of celebrities or models are often altered to "enhance" physical appearance.

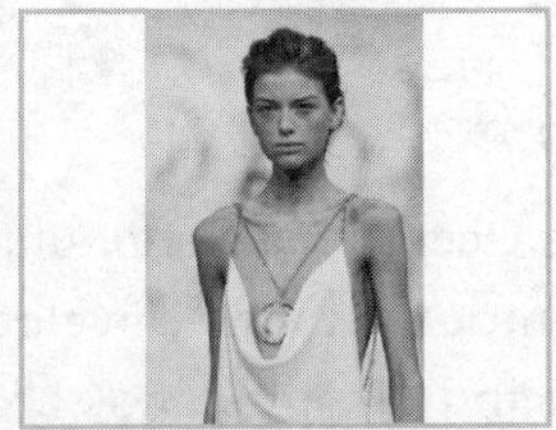

Figure 13.3
Until recently, the "in" look among runway models required extreme emaciation.

III. What Does an Eating Disorder Look Like? (p. 531)

a. Anorexia Nervosa Is a Potentially Deadly Eating Disorder

b. Bulimia Nervosa Is Characterized by Binging and Purging

Key Terms: anorexia nervosa, amenorrhea, bulimia nervosa, binge eating, purging

Instructor Tools: Chapter 13 PPT slides, Chapter 13 PRS Clicker Question slide 3, TAs 292–294, 299–300

Images:

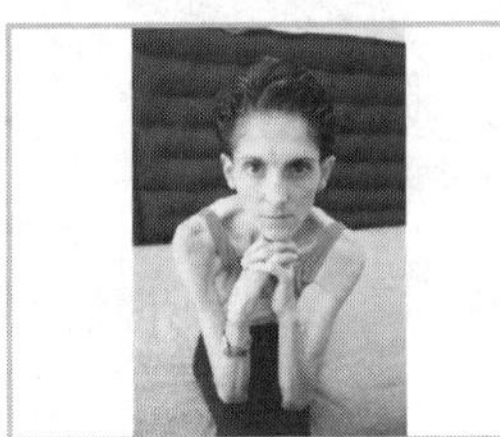

Figure 13.4
Anorexia nervosa.

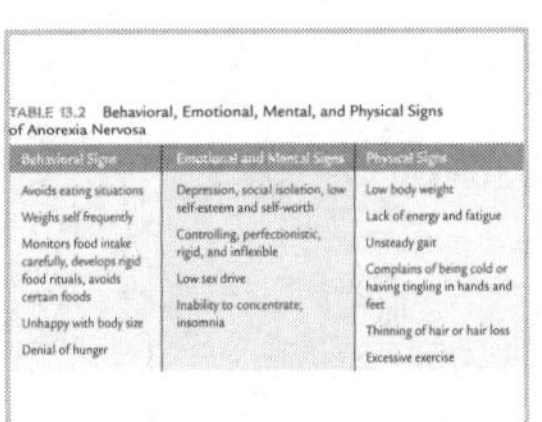

TABLE 13.2 Behavioral, Emotional, Mental, and Physical Signs of Anorexia Nervosa

Behavioral Signs	Emotional and Mental Signs	Physical Signs
Avoids eating situations Weighs self frequently Monitors food intake carefully, develops rigid food rituals, avoids certain foods Unhappy with body size Denial of hunger	Depression, social isolation, low self-esteem and self-worth Controlling, perfectionistic, rigid, and inflexible Low sex drive Inability to concentrate, insomnia	Low body weight Lack of energy and fatigue Unsteady gait Complains of being cold or having tingling in hands and feet Thinning of hair or hair loss Excessive exercise

Table 13.2
Signs of Anorexia Nervosa

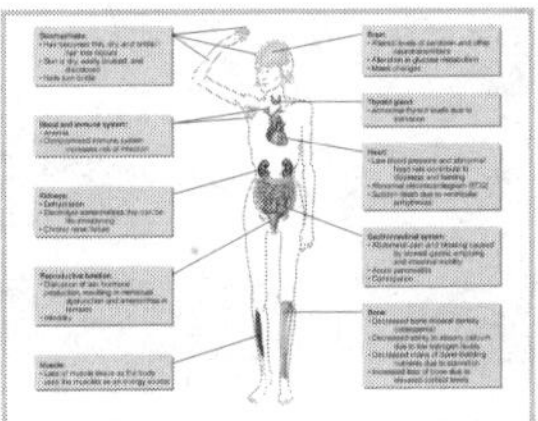

Figure 13.5
Impact of anorexia nervosa on the body.

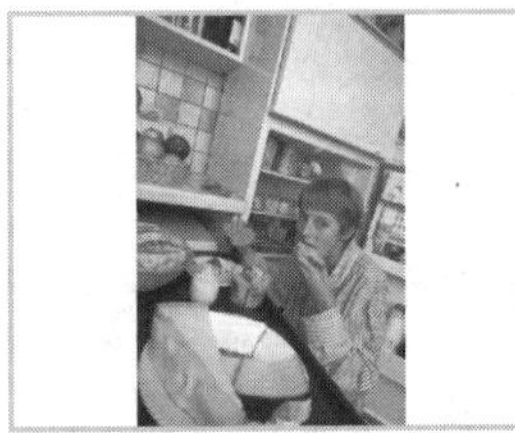

Figure 13.6
Bulimia nervosa.

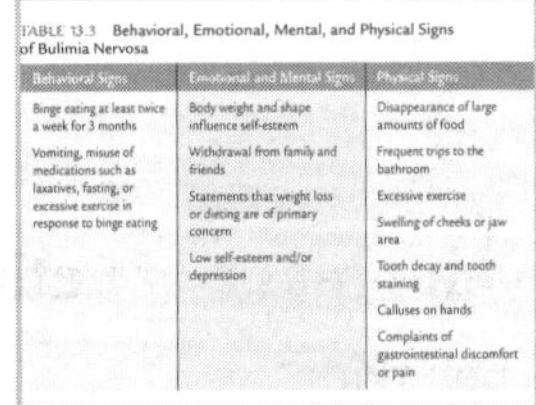

TABLE 13.3 Behavioral, Emotional, Mental, and Physical Signs of Bulimia Nervosa

Behavioral Signs	Emotional and Mental Signs	Physical Signs
Binge eating at least twice a week for 3 months Vomiting, misuse of medications such as laxatives, fasting, or excessive exercise in response to binge eating	Body weight and shape influence self-esteem Withdrawal from family and friends Statements that weight loss or dieting are of primary concern Low self-esteem and/or depression	Disappearance of large amounts of food Frequent trips to the bathroom Excessive exercise Swelling of cheeks or jaw area Tooth decay and tooth staining Calluses on hands Complaints of gastrointestinal discomfort or pain

Table 13.3
Signs of Bulimia Nervosa

Activity:

Have students work in groups to prepare a lecture they might give to adolescents on the dangers of eating disorders. Ask them to include at least four points that could help discourage their audience from this type of behavior. Remind students to support each point they make with specific details. Have each group share its lecture with the class.

IV. What Does Disordered Eating Look Like? (p. 537)

a. Binge-Eating Disorder Can Cause Significant Weight Gain

b. Night-Eating Syndrome Can Lead to Obesity

c. Chronic Dieting Is a Common Pattern of Disordered Eating

Key Terms: Eating Disorders Not Otherwise Specified (EDNOS), binge-eating disorder, night-eating syndrome, chronic dieting, weight cycling

Instructor Tools: Chapter 13 PPT slides, Chapter 13 PRS Clicker Question slide 4, TA 295

Image:

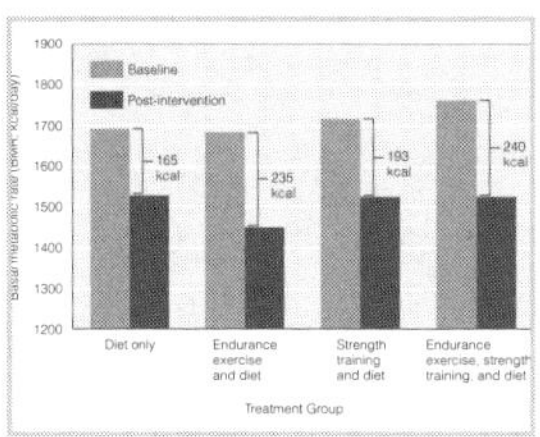

Figure 13.7
Effects of various dieting and exercise strategies on BMR.

V. What Is the Female Athlete Triad? (p. 545)

a. Sports that Emphasize Leanness Increase the Risk for the Female Athlete Triad

b. Three Disorders Characterize the Female Athlete Triad

c. Recognizing and Treating the Female Athlete Triad Can Be Challenging

Key Term: female athlete triad

Instructor Tools: Chapter 13 PPT slides, TA 296

Image:

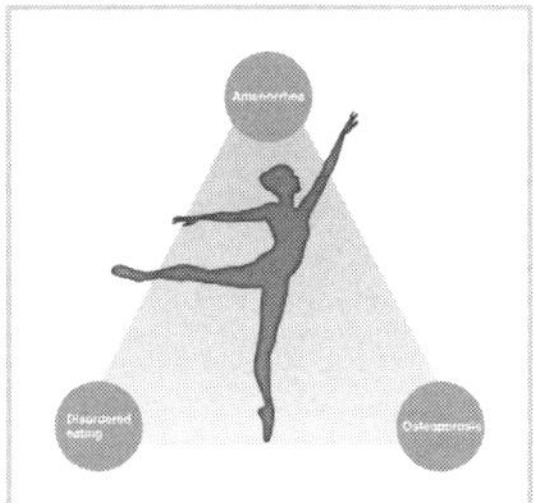

Figure 13.8
The female athlete triad.

Activity:

Ask students to bring to class a magazine that is about a sport they are interested in. Examples would include ski magazines, running magazines, weight lifting magazines, bicycling magazines, etc. Have students work in groups to evaluate the magazines they brought in with regard to the messages that these publications convey. Specifically, ask students to evaluate whether the overall message of these publications is health and fitness or appearance. Discuss what kinds of behavior these publications might encourage, both positive and negative.

VI. What Therapies Work for People with an Eating Disorder? (p. 548)

a. Most Treatment Programs Use a Team Approach

b. Treatment Options Vary According to Several Factors

Instructor Tools: Chapter 13 PPT slides, Chapter 13 PRS Clicker Question slide 5, TA 297

Image:

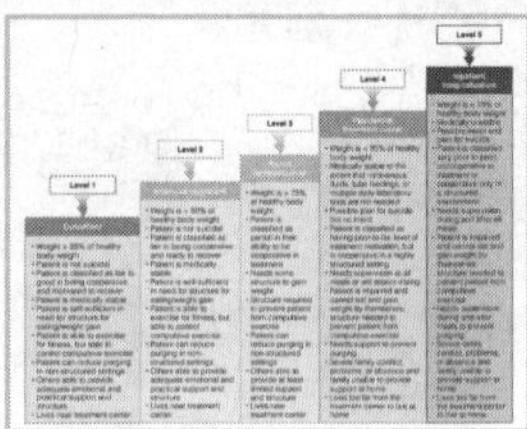

Figure 13.9
Five levels of care for eating disorders.

Activities:

1. Have students research counseling and education resources in the community that help those with eating disorders. Ask students to share their findings with the class.
2. Invite a mental health professional who specializes in treating eating disorders to speak to the class.

VII. How Can We Prevent Eating Disorders and Disordered Eating? (p. 551)

Instructor Tools: Chapter 13 PPT slides

VIII. Additional Chapter 13 Instructor Tools

MyDietAnalysis Activities: Have students keep a journal of food intake for one to three days. As students record their food intake, instruct them to pay attention to the following questions:

a. When do I eat?

b. Do I skip meals often?

c. Where do I eat?

d. Why do I eat?

e. Are there any eating behaviors I'd like to change?

Nutrition Debate Activity: Have students bring in pictures from magazines that demonstrate unrealistic images of body types for men and women. Discuss how the images are similar and how they are different for the different sexes.

Printed TestBank: Pages 182–195 (TestGen Chapter 13)

Quiz Show PowerPoints: Chapter 13

Notes

Food Safety and Technology: Impact on Consumers 14

Chapter at a Glance

I. What Causes Food-Borne Illness?
II. How Can Food-Borne Illness Be Prevented?
III. How Is Food Spoilage Prevented?
IV. What Are Food Additives, and Are They Safe?
V. Do Residues Harm Our Food Supply?

Visual Lecture Outline

I. What Causes Food-Borne Illness? (p. 563)

a. Food-Borne Illness Is Commonly Caused by Microorganisms or Their Toxins

b. Eating Disorders and Disordered Eating Patterns Are Not the Same Thing

Key Terms: food-borne illness, bacteria, viruses, helminth, giardiasis, fungi, prion, toxin, neurotoxins, enterotoxins

Instructor Tools: Chapter 14 PPT slides, Chapter 14 PRS Clicker Question slides 1–3, TAs 301–304, 314–318

Images:

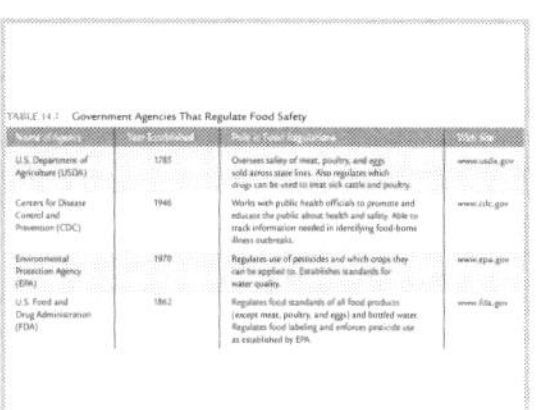

TABLE 14.1 Government Agencies That Regulate Food Safety

Name of Agency	Year Established	Role in Food Regulations	Web Site
U.S. Department of Agriculture (USDA)	1785	Oversees safety of meat, poultry, and eggs sold across state lines. Also regulates which drugs can be used to treat sick cattle and poultry.	www.usda.gov
Centers for Disease Control and Prevention (CDC)	1946	Works with public health officials to promote and educate the public about health and safety. Able to track information needed in identifying food-borne illness outbreaks.	www.cdc.gov
Environmental Protection Agency (EPA)	1970	Regulates use of pesticides and which crops they can be applied to. Establishes standards for water quality.	www.epa.gov
U.S. Food and Drug Administration (FDA)	1862	Regulates food standards of all food products (except meat, poultry, and eggs) and bottled water. Regulates food labeling and enforces pesticide use as established by EPA.	www.fda.gov

Table 14.1
Government Agencies That Regulate Food Safety

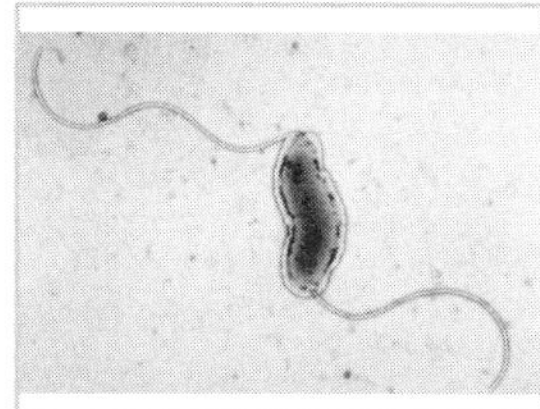

Figure 14.1
Campylobacter jejuni.

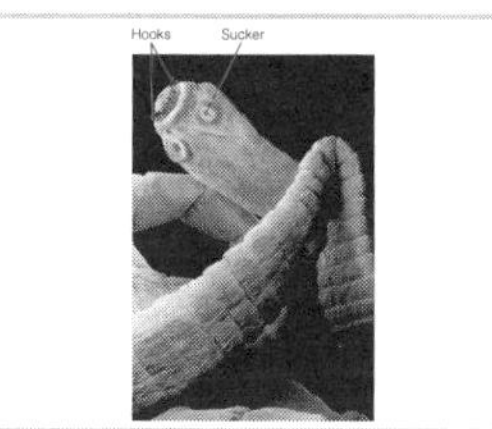

Figure 14.2
Tapeworms.

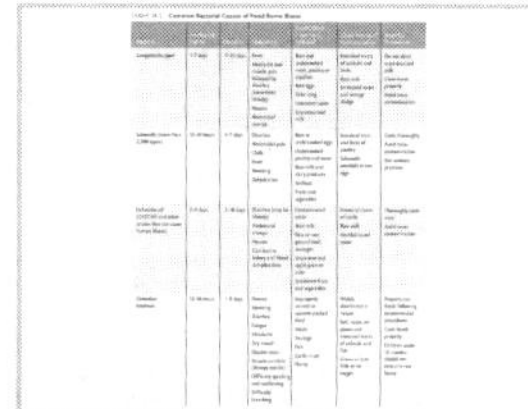

Table 14.2a
Common Bacterial Causes of Food-Borne Illness

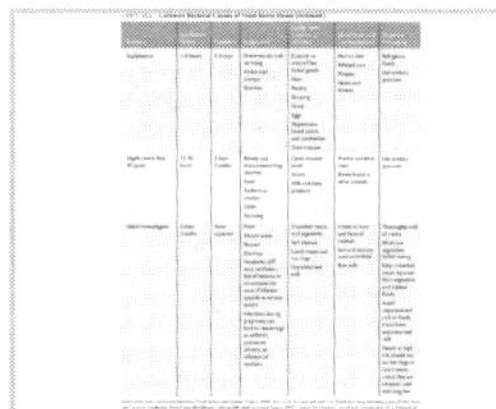

Table 14.2b
Common Bacterial Causes of Food-Borne Illness (*continued*)

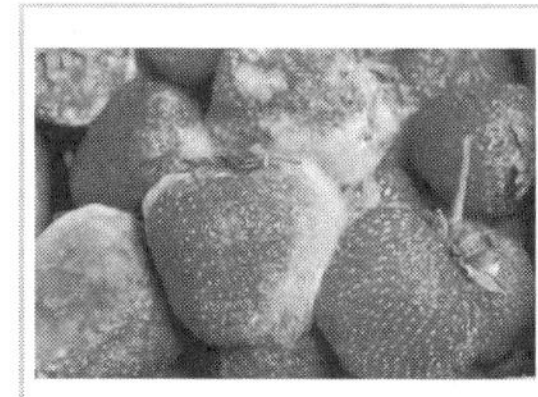

Figure 14.3
Molds.

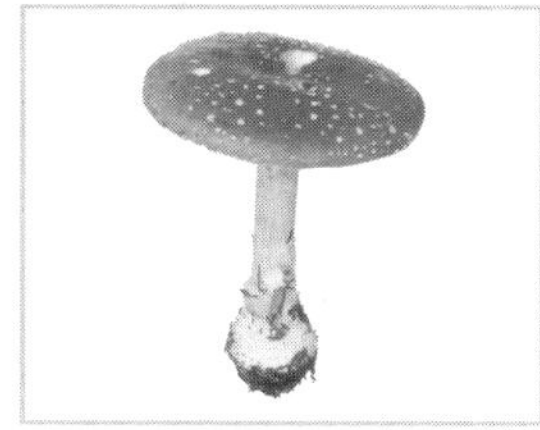

Figure 14.4
Fly agaric mushrooms contain toxins that can cause illness or even death.

II. How Can Food-Borne Illness Be Prevented? (p. 569)

a. When Preparing Foods at Home

b. When Eating Out

c. When Traveling to Other Countries

abc NEWS Lecture Launcher Video:

E. Coli at Home

abc NEWS Video Discussion Questions:

1. Discuss methods of minimizing risk of foodborne illness when purchasing food.
2. Discuss methods of minimizing risk of foodborne illness when preparing food.
3. Discuss methods of minimizing risk of foodborne illness when storing and reheating food.
4. Suggest foods that are most likely to cause food poisoning. Give reasons for your suggestions.
5. Suggest foods that are least likely to cause food poisoning. Give reasons for your suggestions.

Key Terms: cross contamination, biotoxins

Instructor Tools: Chapter 14 PPT slides, Chapter 14 PRS Clicker Question slides 4–5, TAs 305–308, 319

Images:

FIGHT BAC!
SEPARATE
Don't cross-contaminate.
CLEAN
Wash hands and surfaces often.
CHILL
Refrigerate promptly.
COOK
Cook to proper temperatures.
Keep Food Safe From Bacteria™

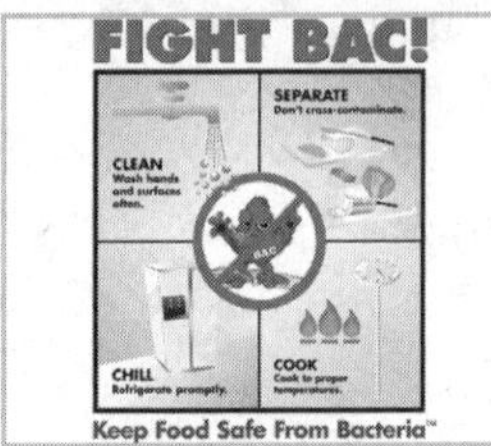

Figure 14.5
The FightBAC! logo is the food safety logo of the USDA.

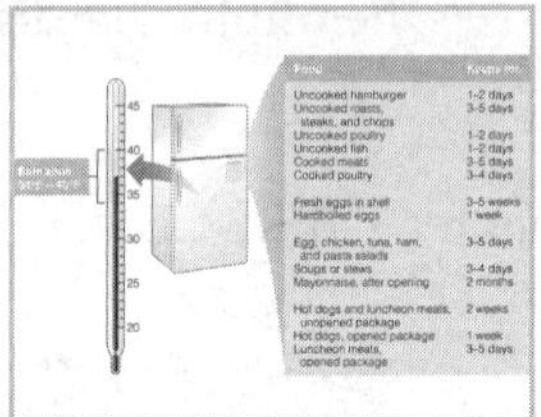

Figure 14.6
It's important to know how long foods will keep.

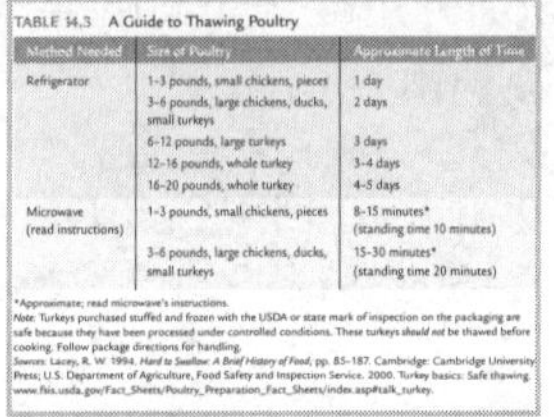

TABLE 14.3 A Guide to Thawing Poultry

Method Needed	Size of Poultry	Approximate Length of Time
Refrigerator	1–3 pounds, small chickens, pieces	1 day
	3–6 pounds, large chickens, ducks, small turkeys	2 days
	6–12 pounds, large turkeys	3 days
	12–16 pounds, whole turkey	3–4 days
	16–20 pounds, whole turkey	4–5 days
Microwave (read instructions)	1–3 pounds, small chickens, pieces	8–15 minutes* (standing time 10 minutes)
	3–6 pounds, large chickens, ducks, small turkeys	15–30 minutes* (standing time 20 minutes)

*Approximate; read microwave's instructions.

Note: Turkeys purchased stuffed and frozen with the USDA or state mark of inspection on the packaging are safe because they have been processed under controlled conditions. These turkeys *should not* be thawed before cooking. Follow package directions for handling.

Sources: Lacey, R. W. 1994. *Hard to Swallow: A Brief History of Food*, pp. 85–187. Cambridge: Cambridge University Press; U.S. Department of Agriculture, Food Safety and Inspection Service. 2000. Turkey basics: Safe thawing. www.fsis.usda.gov/Fact_Sheets/Poultry_Preparation_Fact_Sheets/index.asp#talk_turkey.

Table 14.3
A Guide To Thawing Poultry

Thermy™
"IT'S SAFE TO BITE WHEN THE TEMPERATURE IS RIGHT!"
Temperature Rules!
... for cooking foods at home.
145 °F Beef, lamb & veal steaks & roasts, medium rare (medium—160 °F)
160 °F Ground beef, pork, veal & lamb
Pork chops, ribs & roasts
Egg dishes
165 °F Ground turkey & chicken
Stuffing & casseroles
Leftovers
170 °F Chicken & turkey breasts
180 °F Chicken & turkey
whole bird, legs, thighs & wings
FSIS
USDA Meat and Poultry Hotline
1-888-MPHotline (1-888-674-6854)
TTY: 1-800-256-7072

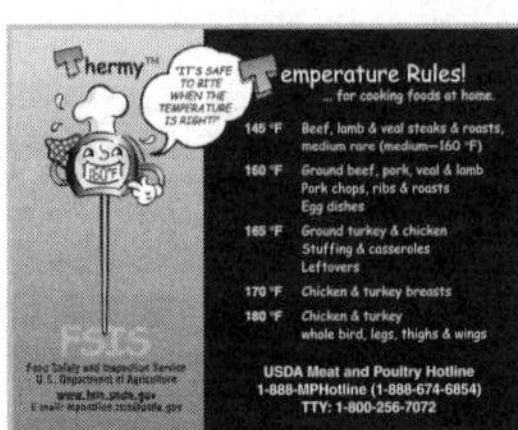

Figure 14.7
The USDA's "Thermy" provides temperature rules for safely cooking foods.

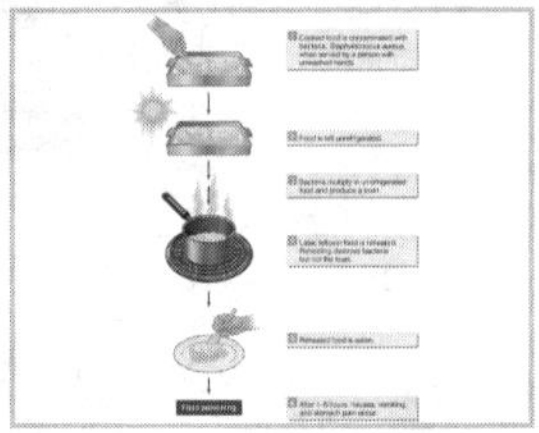

Figure 14.8
Food intoxication can occur long after the microbe itself has been destroyed.

Activities:

1. Have students visit their local supermarket and check 5–10 products in the refrigerated section. Ask students to record the date of their visit, the name of the products they are investigating, and the "use by" or "sell by" date on each product. Ask them to identify any products that have expired dates. Students can share their observations with the class. Discuss the difference between "Use By" and "Sell By" dates.
2. If resources are available, have students take culture samples from kitchen counters, sinks, refrigerator, and freezer in their home. Cultures from hands before and after a thorough washing are also instructive.

III. How Is Food Spoilage Prevented? (p. 578)

a. Natural Methods of Preserving Foods

b. Synthetic Preservative Techniques Improve Food Safety

Key Terms: processed foods, pasteurization, aseptic packaging, food preservatives, BHT (butylated hydroxytoluene), BHA (butylated hydroxyanisole), sulfites, nitrates, nitrites, irradiation, genetic modification, recombinant DNA technology, genetically modified organism (GMO), genetically modified food

Instructor Tools: Chapter 14 PPT slides, TAs 309–311

Images:

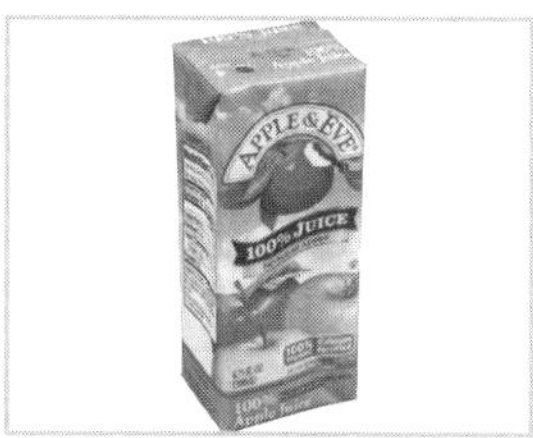

Figure 14.9
Aseptic packaging.

Figure 14.10
Radura—the international symbol of irradiated food.

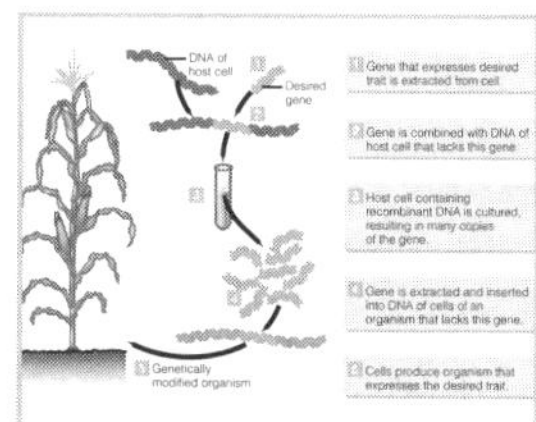

Figure 14.11
Recombinant DNA technology.

Activity:

Have students use the Food Composition Table in Appendix A to compare selected nutrients for foods that are fresh, frozen, canned, or dried. Examples of nutrients that can be compared are:

a total calories

b. vitamin C

c. sodium

d. potassium

e. sugar

Ask students to describe the effects of processing on the nutrient value of the foods we eat.

IV. What Are Food Additives, and Are They Safe? (p. 583)

a. Additives Can Enhance a Food's Taste, Appearance, Safety, or Nutrition

b. Are Food Additives Considered Safe?

Key Terms: food additives, flavoring agents, coaltar, texturizers, stabilizers, thickening agents, emulsifiers, humectants, desiccants, bleaching agents, Generally Recognized as Safe (GRAS)

Instructor Tools: Chapter 14 PPT slides, TAs 320–321

Image:

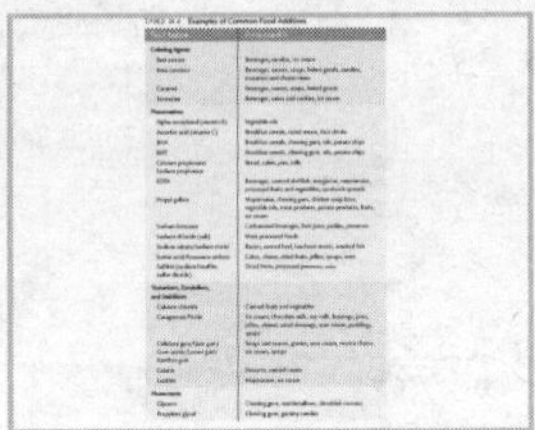

Table 14.4
Examples of Common Food Additives

V. Do Residues Harm Our Food Supply? (p. 586)

a. Persistent Organic Pollutants Can Cause Illness

b. Pesticides Protect Against Crop Losses

c. Growth Hormones Are Injected into Cows to Increase Production of Meat and Milk

Key Terms: residues, persistent organic pollutants (POPs), polychlorinated biphenyls (PCBs), dioxins, pesticides, biopesticides, recombinant bovine growth hormone (rBGH)

Instructor Tools: Chapter 14 PPT slides, Chapter 14 PRS Clicker Question slide 6, TAs 312–313

Images:

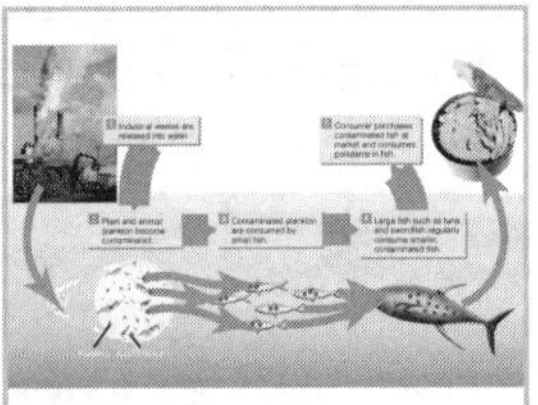

Figure 14.12
Bioaccumulation of persistent organic pollutants in the food supply.

Figure 14.13
The USDA organic seal identifies foods that are at least 95% organic.

Activity:

Invite a representative from the local health department to talk to the class about his or her role in protecting the safety of the food supply. What Therapies Work for People with an Eating Disorder?

VI. Additional Chapter 14 Instructor Tools

MyDietAnalysis Activities: Using the nutritional assessment previously completed, students should identify a processed food that they consumed. Have students evaluate the ingredients list for this food and identify the ingredients they believe are food additives. Ask them to explain the function of each food additive they identify.

Nutrition Debate Activity: Divide students into the following groups: "farmers," "genetic engineers," "GMO opponents," and "general public." Have all students research genetic engineering. When research has been completed, have students present what they learned from the point of view of their group. "Engineers" and "GMO opponents" try to persuade "farmers" to their point of view. "Farmers" decide which option better meets their needs. The "public" presents its needs and decides which group it supports.

Printed TestBank: Pages 196–210 (TestGen Chapter 14)

Quiz Show PowerPoints: Chapter 14

Notes

Nutrition Through the Life Cycle: Pregnancy and the First Year of Life 15

Chapter at a Glance

I. Starting Out Right: Healthful Nutrition in Pregnancy
II. Breastfeeding
III. Infant Nutrition: From Birth to 1 Year

Visual Lecture Outline

I. Starting Out Right: Healthful Nutrition in Pregnancy (p. 602)

a. Is Nutrition Important Before Conception?
b. Why Is Nutrition Important During Pregnancy?
c. How Much Weight Should a Pregnant Woman Gain?
d. What Are a Pregnant Woman's Nutrient Needs?
e. Nutrition-Related Concerns for Pregnant Women

Key Terms: conception (also called *fertilization*), teratogen, trimester, ovulation, zygote, embryo, spontaneous abortion (also called *miscarriage*), placenta, fetus, umbilical cord, neonatal, gestation, low birth weight, preterm, small for gestational age (SGA), neural tube, anencephaly, spina bifida, amniotic fluid, urinary tract infection, morning sickness, pica, gestational diabetes, preeclampsia, fetal alcohol syndrome (FAS), fetal alcohol effects (FAE)

Instructor Tools: Chapter 15 PPT slides, Chapter 15 PRS Clicker Question slides 1–2, TAs 324–330, 336–337

Images:

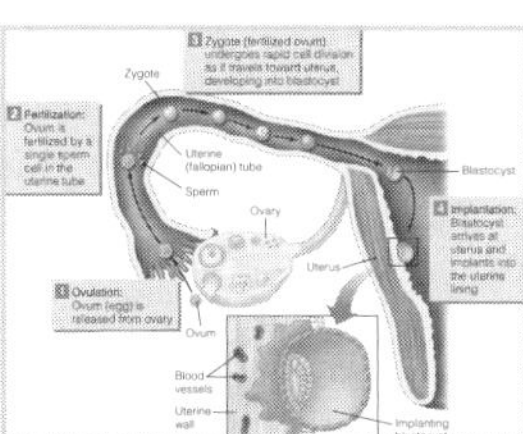

Figure 15.1
Ovulation, conception, and implantation.

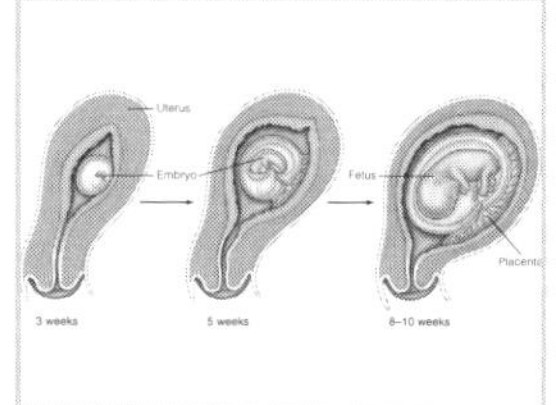

Figure 15.2
Human embryonic development during the first ten weeks.

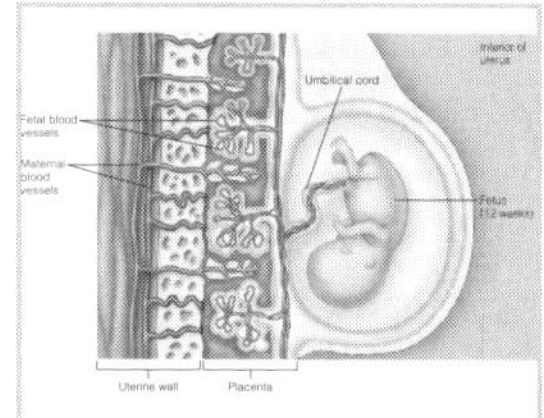

Figure 15.3
Placental development.

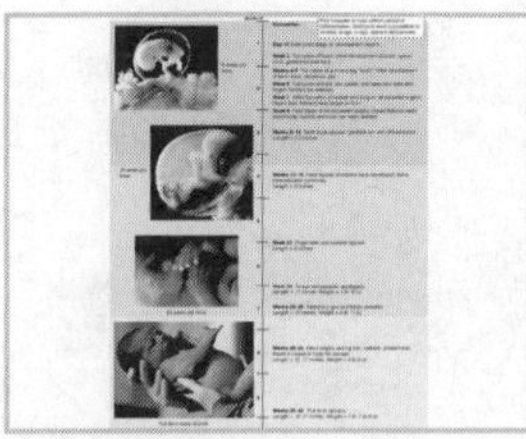

Figure 15.4
A timeline of embryonic and fetal development.

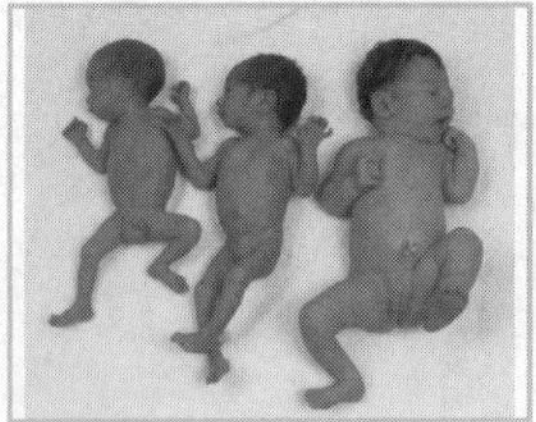

Figure 15.5
A healthy 2-day-old infant (right) compared with two low-birth-weight infants.

TABLE 15.1 Recommended Weight Gain for Women During Pregnancy

Pre-Pregnancy Weight Status	Body Mass Index (kg/m^2)	Recommended Weight Gain (lb)
Normal	18.5–25.0	25–35
Underweight	<18.5	28–40
Overweight	25.1–29.9	15–25
Obese	≥30.0	No more than 15

Table 15.1
Recommended Weight Gain for Women During Pregnancy

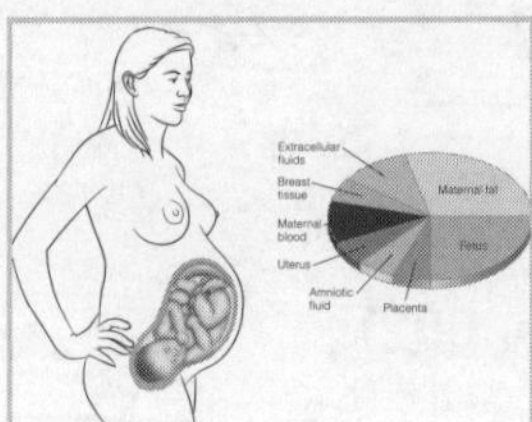

Figure 15.6
Distribution of weight gained during pregnancy.

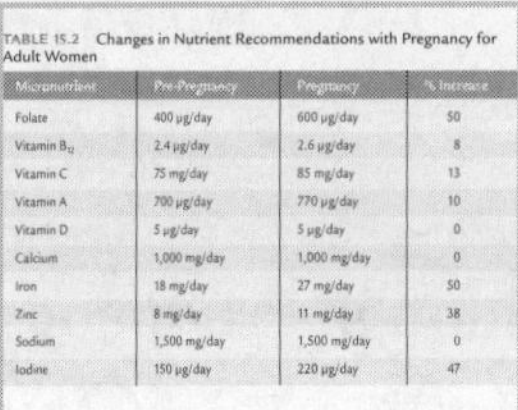

TABLE 15.2 Changes in Nutrient Recommendations with Pregnancy for Adult Women

Micronutrient	Pre-Pregnancy	Pregnancy	% Increase
Folate	400 µg/day	600 µg/day	50
Vitamin B_{12}	2.4 µg/day	2.6 µg/day	8
Vitamin C	75 mg/day	85 mg/day	13
Vitamin A	700 µg/day	770 µg/day	10
Vitamin D	5 µg/day	5 µg/day	0
Calcium	1,000 mg/day	1,000 mg/day	0
Iron	18 mg/day	27 mg/day	50
Zinc	8 mg/day	11 mg/day	38
Sodium	1,500 mg/day	1,500 mg/day	0
Iodine	150 µg/day	220 µg/day	47

Table 15.2
Changes in Nutrient Recommendations With Pregnancy for Adult Women

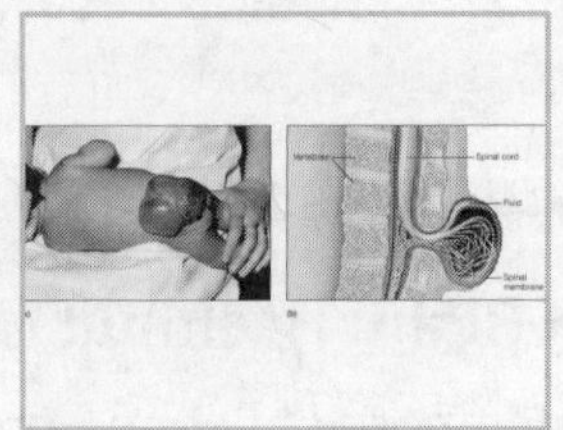

Figure 15.7
Spina bifida, a common neural tube defect.

Activity:

Divide students into groups and have them prepare a list of birth defects that may be related to nutrition. For each birth defect, ask students to suggest ways to prevent it and at what point in the pregnancy (or before conception) the greatest impact is possible.

II. Breastfeeding (p. 618)

a. How Does Lactation Occur?

b. What Are a Breastfeeding Woman's Nutrient Needs?

c. Getting Real About Breastfeeding: Pros and Cons

abc NEWS **Lecture Launcher Video:**

Breast Feeding

abc NEWS **Video Discussion Questions:**

1. Do you believe bottle-fed babies are "harmed"? Give reasons to support your opinion.
2. Should the government enact stronger laws to facilitate breastfeeding in the work place? Why or why not?
3. Are you comfortable with breastfeeding in a public setting? Why or why not?

Key Terms: lactation, colostrum, sudden infant death syndrome (SIDS)

Instructor Tools: Chapter 15 PPT slides, Chapter 15 PRS Clicker Question slides 3–4, TAs 331–332

Images:

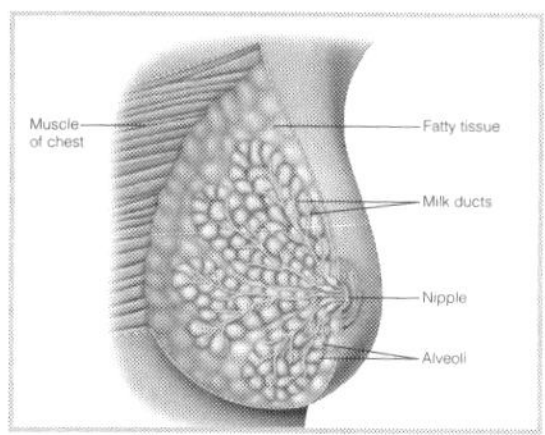

Figure 15.8
Anatomy of the breast.

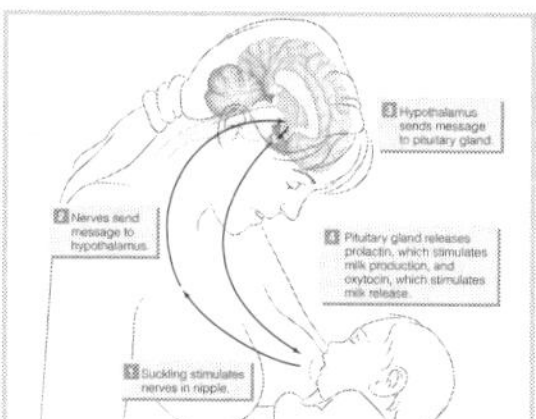

Figure 15.9
Suckling stimulus for breastfeeding.

Activity:

Have each student take a poll of at least five mothers. Have them ask each mother whether or not she breastfed her infant(s) and why she made the decision she did. Have them note the age of each mother they poll. In class, discuss the findings.

III. Infant Nutrition: From Birth to 1 Year (p. 626)

a. Typical Infant Growth and Activity Patterns
b. Nutrient Needs for Infants
c. What *Not* to Feed an Infant
d. Nutrition-Related Concerns for Infants

Key Terms: colic, dental caries

Instructor Tools: Chapter 15 PPT slides, Chapter 15 PRS Clicker Question slide 5, TAs 333–335

Images:

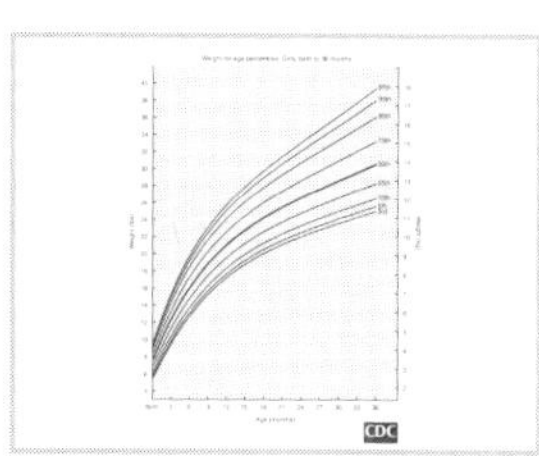

Figure 15.10
A weight-for-age growth chart.

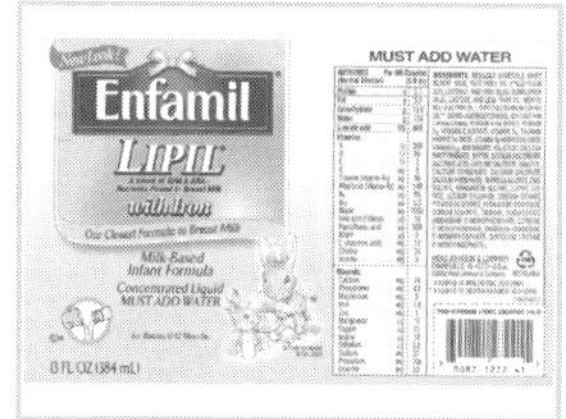

Figure 15.11
An infant formula label.

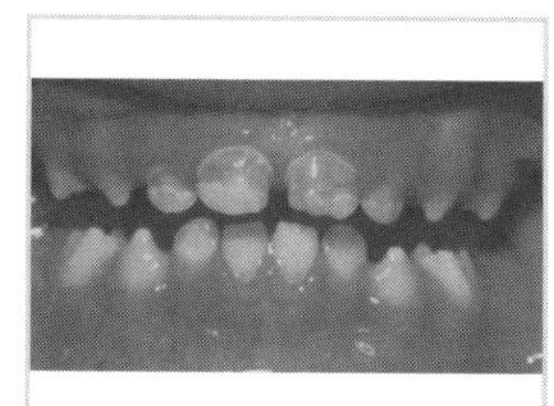

Figure 15.12
Nursing bottle syndrome.

Activities:

1. Have students bring in food labels of various formulas. Many of these are available on the Internet or can be obtained by reading a food label in the grocery store. Make sure different types of formulas are investigated: modified cow milk, soy based, lactose free, etc. Have students note the differences between the formulas and breast milk.
2. Have students use the weight-for-age growth chart in Figure 15.10 on page 627 to evaluate the weight gain of the following girls.

	Age (mos)	0	3	6	9	12
Girl A	Weight (lbs)	8.1	13.0	17.0	20.0	22.6
Girl B	Weight (lbs)	6.0	9.8	12.4	14.9	16.8

IV. Additional Chapter 15 Instructor Tools

MyDietAnalysis Activity: Pregnant women need to be especially careful to consume adequate amounts of folate, vitamin B_{12}, vitamin C, vitamin D, calcium, iron, and zinc. Using the nutritional assessment previously completed, students should note their own intake of these nutrients. Ask students to compare their own intake to the recommended intakes for pregnant women. If any of their intakes are below recommendations, have them suggest ways to reach the appropriate levels for pregnant women.

Nutrition Debate Activity: Have students survey businesses in the community to find out their policy on breastfeeding. They can also survey their peers and other members of the community to find out how individuals view breastfeeding in public and in the workplace. Discuss the findings in class and debate the pros and cons of this issue.

Printed TestBank: Pages 211–224 (TestGen Chapter 15)

MyDietAnalysis Online Assignment: Rita and Ben: Pregnancy and Lactation

Quiz Show PowerPoints: Chapter 15

Nutrition Through the Life Cycle: Childhood to Late Adulthood 16

Chapter at a Glance

I. Nutrition for Toddlers, Ages 1–3 Years
II. Nutrition for Children, Ages 4–13 Years
III. Nutrition for Adolescents, Ages 14–18 Years
IV. Nutrition for Older Adults, Ages 65 Years and Older

Visual Lecture Outline

I. Nutrition for Toddlers, Ages 1–3 Years (p. 642)

a. What Are a Toddler's Nutrient Needs?

b. Encouraging Nutritious Choices with Toddlers

c. Nutrition-Related Concerns for Toddlers

Instructor Tools: Chapter 16 PPT slides, Chapter 16 PRS Clicker Question slides 1–2, TAs 338–339, 350

Images:

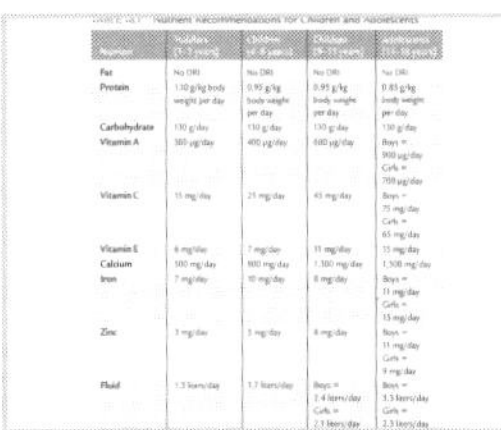

Table 16.1
Nutrient Recommendations for Children and Adolescents

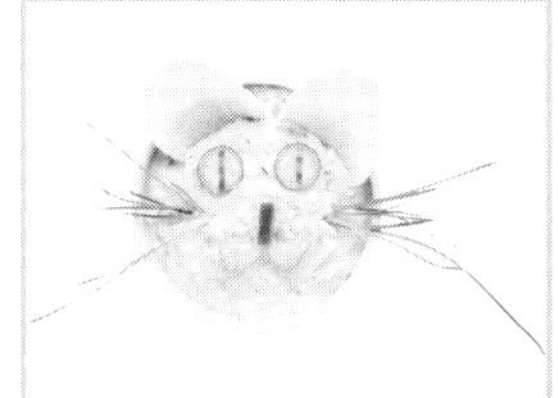

Figure 16.1
Most toddlers are delighted by food prepared in a fun way.

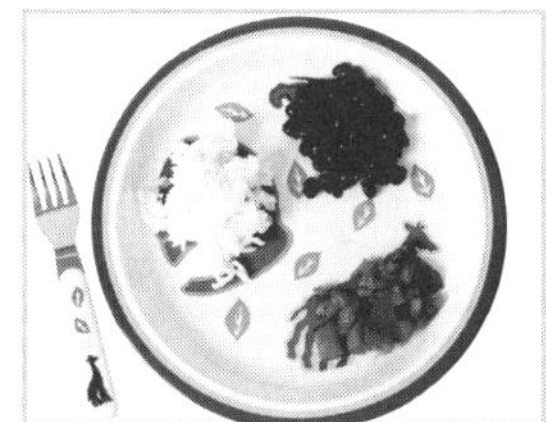

Figure 16.2
Portion sizes for preschoolers.

II. Nutrition for Children, Ages 4–13 Years (p. 648)

a. What Are a Child's Nutrient Needs?

b. Encouraging Nutritious Food Choices with Children

c. Nutrition-Related Concerns for Children

Key Terms: at risk for overweight (childhood), overweight (childhood)

Instructor Tools: Chapter 16 PPT slides, Chapter 16 PRS Clicker Question slide 3, TAs 340–344

Images:

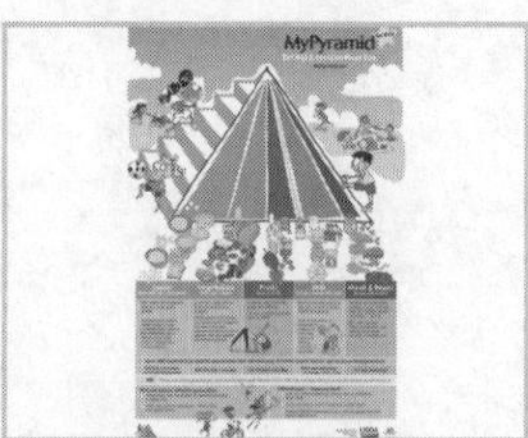

Figure 16.3
MyPyramid for Kids.

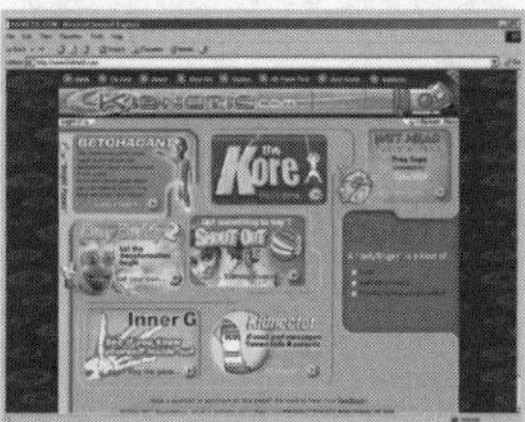
Figure 16.4
Kidnetic.com

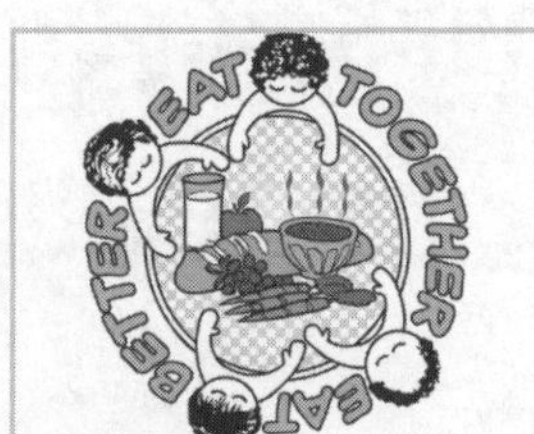

Figure 16.5
"Eat Better, Eat Together."

Activities:

1. Have students watch one hour of Saturday morning children's television and keep track of non-nutritious versus nutritious food commercials. Discuss the marketing strategies used to attract children's attention.
2. Have students work in groups to design simple games (for example, card games, board games, etc.) for teaching children about nutrition. Different student groups can be asked to target a specific age group. Possible age groups include toddlers, children ages 4–7, children ages 8–13, and adolescents.

III. Nutrition for Adolescents, Ages 14–18 Years (p. 655)

a. Adolescent Growth and Activity Patterns
b. What Are an Adolescent's Nutrient Needs?
c. Encouraging Nutritious Food Choices with Adolescents
d. Nutrition-Related Concerns for Adolescents

abc NEWS **Lecture Launcher Video:**

Obesity in Children

abc NEWS **Video Discussion Questions:**

1. Discuss strategies that can help prevent obesity in children.
2. Do you believe childhood obesity is more of a physical problem or a psychological problem? Explain.
3. Discuss potential reasons for the observation that obese parents are more likely to have obese children. How can this cycle be reversed?

Key Terms: puberty, menarche, epiphyseal plates

Instructor Tools: Chapter 16 PPT slides, TA 345

Image:

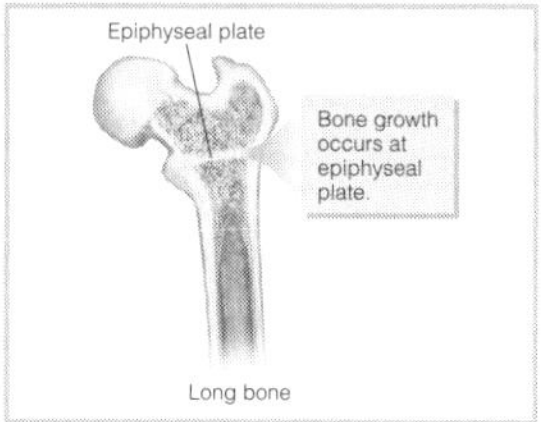

Figure 16.6
Skeletal growth ceases once closure of the epiphyseal plates occurs.

Activity:

Have students visit a high school in their community and determine if there is a vending machine on the premises. When a vending machine (or machines) is present, ask the students to make a note of the foods and/or beverages that are in the machine(s) and evaluate their nutritional quality. Ask them to make suggestions for improvements.

IV. Nutrition for Older Adults, Age 65 Years and Older (p. 660)

a. What Physiologic Changes Accompany Aging?

b. What Are an Older Adult's Nutrient Needs?

c. Nutrition-Related Concerns for Older Adults

Instructor Tools: Chapter 16 PPT slides, Chapter 16 PRS Clicker Question slides 4–5, TAs 346–349, 351–352

Images:

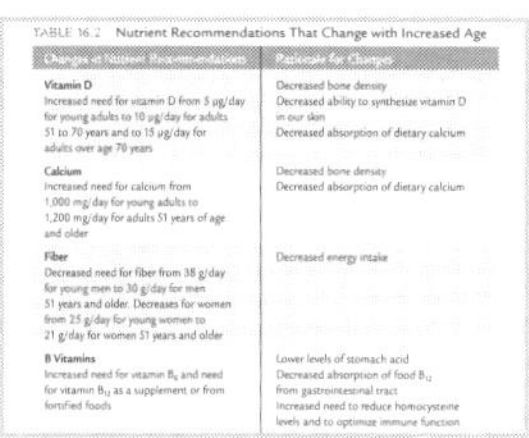

TABLE 16.2 Nutrient Recommendations That Change with Increased Age

Changes in Nutrient Recommendations	Rationale for Changes
Vitamin D Increased need for vitamin D from 5 μg/day for young adults to 10 μg/day for adults 51 to 70 years and to 15 μg/day for adults over age 70 years	Decreased bone density Decreased ability to synthesize vitamin D in our skin Decreased absorption of dietary calcium
Calcium Increased need for calcium from 1,000 mg/day for young adults to 1,200 mg/day for adults 51 years of age and older	Decreased bone density Decreased absorption of dietary calcium
Fiber Decreased need for fiber from 38 g/day for young men to 30 g/day for men 51 years and older. Decreases for women from 25 g/day for young women to 21 g/day for women 51 years and older	Decreased energy intake
B Vitamins Increased need for vitamin B_6 and need for vitamin B_{12} as a supplement or from fortified foods	Lower levels of stomach acid Decreased absorption of food B_{12} from gastrointestinal tract Increased need to reduce homocysteine levels and to optimize immune function

Table 16.2
Nutrient Recommendations That Change with Increased Age

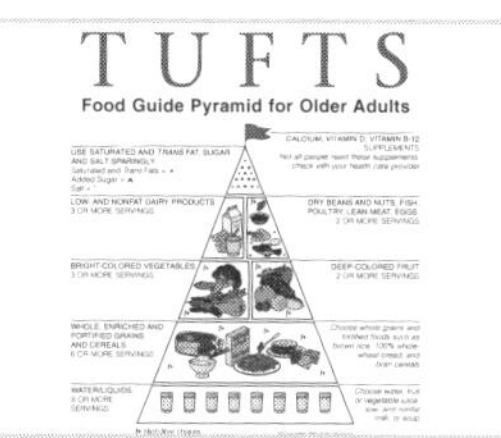

Figure 16.7
The Tufts Modified Food Guide Pyramid for Older (70+) Adults.

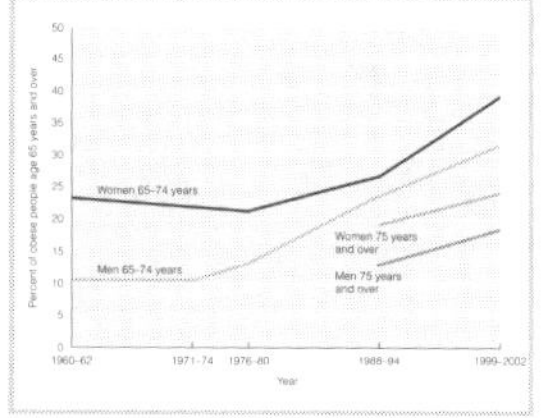

Figure 16.8
Obesity is becoming more common in the U.S. elderly population.

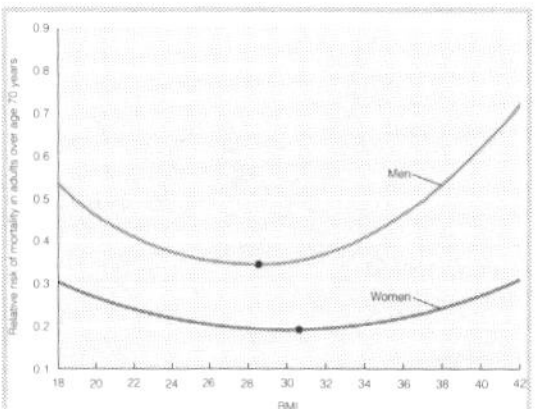

Figure 16.9
The effects of underweight and overweight on mortality in the elderly.

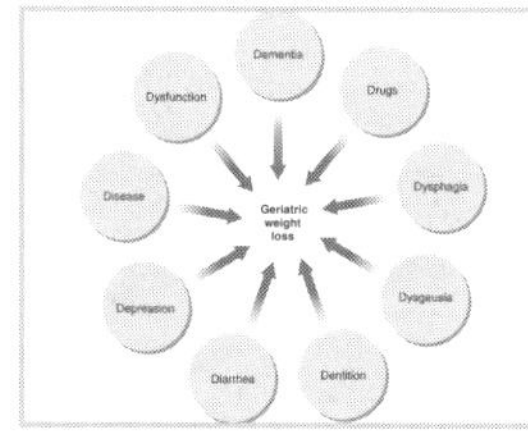

Figure 16.10
The nine Ds of geriatric weight loss.

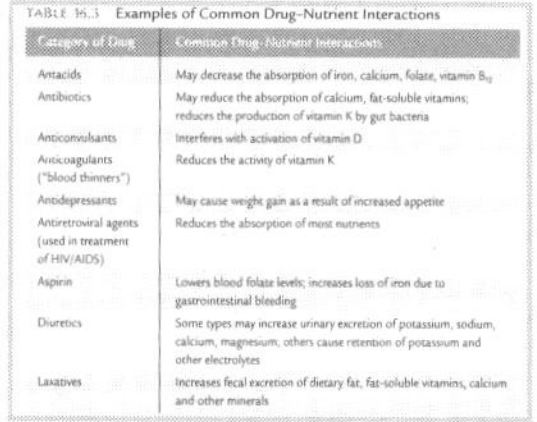

TABLE 16.3 Examples of Common Drug-Nutrient Interactions

Category of Drug	Common Drug-Nutrient Interactions
Antacids	May decrease the absorption of iron, calcium, folate, vitamin B_{12}
Antibiotics	May reduce the absorption of calcium, fat-soluble vitamins; reduces the production of vitamin K by gut bacteria
Anticonvulsants	Interferes with activation of vitamin D
Anticoagulants ("blood thinners")	Reduces the activity of vitamin K
Antidepressants	May cause weight gain as a result of increased appetite
Antiretroviral agents (used in treatment of HIV/AIDS)	Reduces the absorption of most nutrients
Aspirin	Lowers blood folate levels; increases loss of iron due to gastrointestinal bleeding
Diuretics	Some types may increase urinary excretion of potassium, sodium, calcium, magnesium; others cause retention of potassium and other electrolytes
Laxatives	Increases fecal excretion of dietary fat, fat-soluble vitamins, calcium and other minerals

Table 16.3
Common Drug-Nutrient Interactions

Activity:

Have students interview an elderly person about food intake on the previous day and analyze that person's intake according to the government recommendations for the elderly. In small groups, have students compare which food groups were commonly eaten in lower than recommended amounts and which in greater than recommended amounts.

V. Additional Chapter 16 Instructor Tools

MyDietAnalysis Activity: Have students choose a lunch from a school lunch menu to evaluate using their diet analysis software. Ask them to note which nutrients are low and which are high. They should then evaluate the nutrient density of this meal and suggest improvements.

Nutrition Debate Activity: Ask students to redesign one day of their previously completed food journal to reflect a 35% reduction in caloric intake. Discuss in class how difficult students believe it would be to maintain an energy intake at this level.

Printed TestBank: Pages 225–237 (TestGen Chapter 16)

MyDietAnalysis Online Assignment: Hannah: 9-Year-Old's Diet

Quiz Show PowerPoints: Chapter 16

In Depth: Global Nutrition

Chapter at a Glance

I. Malnutrition in the Developing World
II. Malnutrition in the United States
III. What Can Be Done to Relieve Malnutrition?

Visual Lecture Outline

I. Malnutrition in the Developing World (p. 681)

a. What Causes Hunger in Developing Nations?

b. What Health Problems Result from Undernutrition?

c. Why Is Obesity a Growing Problem in Developing Nations?

Key Terms: malnutrition, undernutrition, overnutrition, wasting, stunting, famine, overpopulated, cash crops, nutrition transition

Instructor Tools: In Depth: Global PPT slides, In Depth: Global PRS Clicker Questions slides 1–4, TAs 353–354

Images:

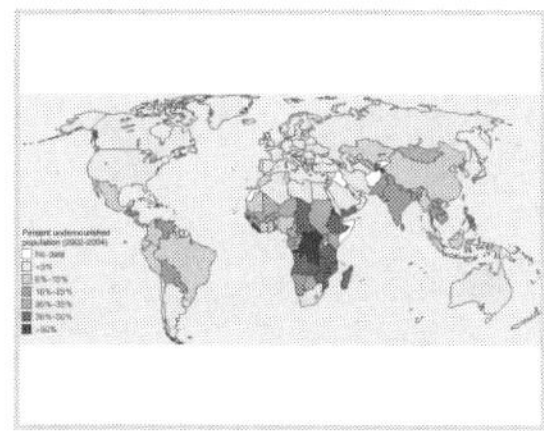

Figure 1
Map of undernutrition.

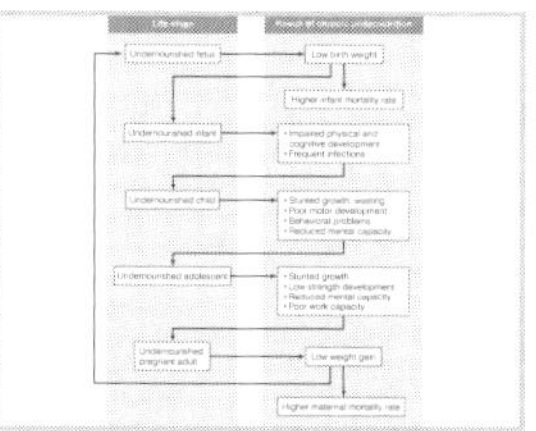

Figure 2
Acute and long-term effects of malnutrition throughout the lifecycle.

II. Malnutrition in the United States (p. 685)

Key Term: food insecurity

Instructor Tools: In Depth: Global PPT slides, TA 355

Image:

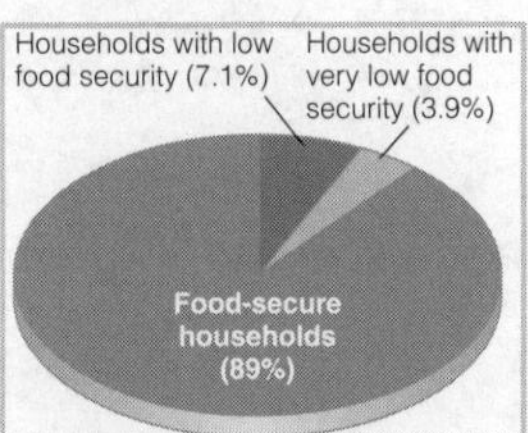

Figure 3
Food security status of U.S. households in 2005.

Activities:

1. Have students work in groups to research and identify current problem areas for hunger world-wide. Ask them to investigate the cause of the problem and whether or not there has been an adequate response by relief agencies.
2. Working in groups, have students develop a monthly shopping list with a budget of $155—the maximum monthly allowable food stamp allotment for one person (based on October 1, 2006-September 30, 2007 guidelines).

III. What Can Be Done to Relieve Malnutrition? (p. 685)

a. Global Solutions

b. Local Solutions

c. Get Involved!

Key Terms: sustainable agriculture, transgenic crops

Instructor Tools: In Depth: Global PPT slides, In Depth: Global PRS Clicker Questions slide 5, TA 356

Image:

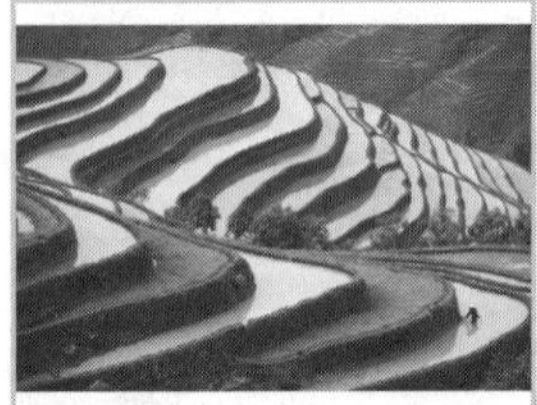

Figure 4
Terracing sloped land to avoid soil erosion.

Activity:

Ask students to volunteer in a local program that provides meals to the hungry. Have them share their experience with the class.

IV. Additional In Depth: Global Nutrition Instructor Tools

MyDietAnalysis Activity: Using the food-stamp shopping list from the second Activity in the Malnutrition in the U.S. section, have students plan a breakfast, lunch, or dinner. Ask them to analyze the meals using their MyDietAnalysis software and note which nutrients are adequate, which are high, and which are low.

Printed TestBank: Pages 238–241 (TestGen In Depth: Global Nutrition)

Notes

Teaching Tips for First-Time Instructors and Adjunct Professors

How to Be an Effective Teacher

(From David Royse, *Teaching Tips for College and University Instructors: A Practical Guide,* published by Allyn & Bacon, Boston, MA. © 2001 by Pearson Education, Inc. Adapted by permission of the publisher.)

A look at fifty years of research "on the way teachers teach and learners learn" reveals five broad principles of good teaching practice (Chickering and Gamson, 1987).

Five Principles of Good Teaching Practice

1. **Frequent student-faculty contact:** Faculty who are concerned about their students and their progress and who are perceived to be easy to talk to, serve to motivate and keep students involved.

   Things you can do to apply this principle:

   - Attend events sponsored by students.
   - Serve as a mentor or advisor to students.
   - Keep "open" or "drop-in" office hours.

2. **The encouragement of cooperation among students:** There is a wealth of research indicating that students benefit from the use of small-group and peer-learning instructional approaches.

   Things you can do to apply this principle:

   - Have students share in class their interests and backgrounds.
   - Create small groups to work on projects together.
   - Encourage students to study together.

3. **Prompt feedback:** Learning theory research has consistently shown that the quicker the feedback, the greater the learning.

   Things you can do to apply this principle:

   - Return quizzes and exams by the next class meeting.
   - Return homework within one week.
   - Provide students with detailed comments on their written papers.

4. **Emphasize time on task:** This principle refers to the amount of actual involvement with the material being studied and applies, obviously, to the way the instructor uses classroom instructional time. Faculty need good time-management skills.

   Things you can do to apply this principle:

   - Require students who miss classes to make up lost work.
   - Require students to rehearse before making oral presentations.
   - Don't let class breaks stretch out too long.

5. **Communicating high expectations:** The key here is not to make the course impossibly difficult but to have goals that can be attained as long as individual learners stretch and work hard, going beyond what they already know.

   Things you can do to apply this principle:

   - Communicate your expectations orally and in writing at the beginning of the course.
   - Explain the penalties for students who turn work in late.
   - Identify excellent work by students; display exemplars if possible.

Tips for Thriving

CREATING AN INCLUSIVE CLASSROOM

How do you model an open, accepting attitude within your classroom where students will feel it is safe to engage in give-and-take discussions? First, view students as individuals instead of representatives of separate and distinct groups. Cultivate a climate that is respectful of diverse viewpoints, and don't allow ridicule, or defamatory or hurtful remarks. Try to encourage everyone in the class to participate, and be alert to showing favoritism.

Planning Your Course

(From David Royse, *Teaching Tips for College and University Instructors: A Practical Guide,* published by Allyn & Bacon, Boston, MA. © 2001 by Pearson Education, Inc. Adapted by permission of the publisher.)

Constructing the syllabus: The syllabus should clearly communicate course objectives, assignments, required readings, and grading policies. Think of the syllabus as a stand-alone document. Those students who miss the first or second meeting of a class should be able to learn most of what they need to know about the requirements of the course from reading the syllabus. Start by collecting syllabi from colleagues who have recently taught the course you will be teaching and look for common threads and themes.

Problems to avoid: One mistake commonly made by educators teaching a course for the first time is that they may have rich and intricate visions of how they want students to demonstrate comprehension and synthesis of the material, but they somehow fail to convey this information to those enrolled. Check your syllabus to make sure your expectations have been fully articulated. Be very specific. Avoid vaguely worded instructions that can be misinterpreted.

Tips for Thriving

VISUAL QUALITY

Students today are highly visual learners, so you should give special emphasis to the visual quality of the materials you provide to students. Incorporate graphics into your syllabus and other handouts. Color code your materials so materials for different sections of the course are on different-colored papers. Such visuals are likely to create a perception among students that you are contemporary.

Your First Class

(From Richard E. Lyons, Marcella L. Kysilka, & George E. Pawlas, *The Adjunct Professor's Guide to Success: Surviving and Thriving In The Classroom,* published by Allyn & Bacon, Boston, MA. © 1999 by Pearson Education, Inc. Adapted by permission of the publisher.)

Success in achieving a great start is almost always directly attributable to the quality and quantity of planning that has been invested by the course professor. If the first meeting of your class is to be successful, you should strive to achieve seven distinct goals.

Seven Goals for a Successful First Meeting

1. **Create a positive first impression:** Renowned communications consultant Roger Ailes claims you have fewer than 10 seconds to create a positive image of yourself. Students are greatly influenced by the visual component; therefore, you must look the part of the professional professor. Dress as you would for a professional job interview. Greet each student entering the room. Be approachable and genuine.
2. **Introduce yourself effectively:** Communicate to students who you are and why you are credible as the teacher of the course. Seek to establish your approachability by "building common ground," such as stating your understanding of students' hectic lifestyles or their common preconceptions toward the subject matter.
3. **Clarify the goals and expectations:** Make a transparency of each page of the syllabus for display on an overhead projector and, using a cover sheet, expose each section as you explain it. Provide clarification and elicit questions.
4. **Conduct an activity that introduces students to each other:** Students' chances of being able to complete a course effectively are enhanced if each comes to perceive the classmates as a "support network." The small amount of time you invest in an icebreaker will help create a positive classroom atmosphere and pay additional dividends throughout the term.
5. **Learn students' names:** A student who is regularly addressed by name feels more valued, is invested more effectively in classroom discussion, and will approach the professor with questions and concerns.
6. **Whet students' appetite for the course material:** The textbook adopted for the course is critical to your success. Your first meeting should include a review of its approach, features, and sequencing. Explain to students what percentage of class tests will be derived from material from the textbook.
7. **Reassure students of the value of the course:** At the close of your first meeting reassure students that the course will be a valuable learning experience and a wise investment of their time. Review the reasons why the course is a good investment: important and relevant content, interesting classmates, and a dynamic classroom environment.

Strategies for Teaching and Learning

(From David Royse, *Teaching Tips for College and University Instructors: A Practical Guide,* published by Allyn & Bacon, Boston, MA. © 2001 by Pearson Education, Inc. Adapted by permission of the publisher.)

Team learning: The essential features of this small-group learning approach, developed originally for use in large college classrooms, are (1) relatively permanent heterogeneous task groups; (2) grading based on a combination of individual performance, group performance, and peer evaluation; (3) organization of the course so that the majority of class time is spent on small-group activities; and (4) a six-step instructional process similar to the following model:

1. Individual study of material outside of the class is assigned.
2. Individual testing is used (multiple-choice questions over homework at the beginning of class).
3. Groups discuss their answers and then are given a group test of the same items. They then get immediate feedback (answers).
4. Groups may prepare written appeals of items.
5. Feedback is given from instructor.
6. An application-oriented activity is assigned (e.g., a problem to be solved requiring input from all group members).

If you plan to use team learning in your class, inform students at the beginning of the course of your intentions to do so and explain the benefits of small-group learning. Foster group cohesion by sitting groups together and letting them choose "identities" such as a team name or slogan. You will need to structure and supervise the groups and ensure that the projects build on newly acquired learning. Make the projects realistic and interesting and ensure that they are adequately structured so that each member's contribution is 25 percent. Students should be given criteria by which they can assess and evaluate the contributions of their peers on a project-by-project basis (Michaelsen, 1994).

Tips for Thriving

ACTIVE LEARNING AND LECTURING

Lecturing is one of the most time-honored teaching methods, but does it have a place in an active learning environment? There are times when lecturing can be effective. Think about the following when planning a lecture:

Build interest: Capture your students' attention by leading off with an anecdote or cartoon.

Maximize understanding and retention: Use brief handouts and demonstrations as a visual backup to enable your students to see as well as hear.

Involve students during the lecture: Interrupt the lecture occasionally to challenge students to answer spot quiz questions.

Reinforce the lecture: Give students a self-scoring review test at the end of the lecture.

Grading and Assessment Techniques

(From Philip C. Wankat, *The Effective, Efficient Professor: Teaching Scholarship and Service,* published by Allyn & Bacon, Boston, MA. © 2002 by Pearson Education, Inc. Adapted by permission of the publisher.)

Philosophy of grading: Develop your own philosophy of grading by picturing in your mind the performance of typical A students, B students, and so on. Try different grading methods until you find one that fits your philosophy and is reasonably fair. Always look closely at students on grade borders—take into account personal factors if the group is small. Be consistent with or slightly more generous than the procedure outlined in your syllabus.

Criterion grading: Professor Philip Wankat writes: "I currently use a form of criterion grading for my sophomore and junior courses. I list the scores in the syllabus that will guarantee the students A's, B's, and so forth. For example, a score of 85 to 100 guarantees an A; 75 to 85, a B; 65 to 75, a C; and 55 to 65, a D. If half the class gets above 85% they all get an A. This reduces competition and allows students to work together and help each other. The standard grade gives students something to aim for and tells them exactly what their grade is at any time. For students whose net scores are close to the borders at the end of the course, I look at other factors before deciding a final grade such as attendance."

Tips for Thriving:

RESULT FEEDBACK

As stated earlier, feedback on results is the most effective of motivating factors. Anxious students are especially hungry for positive feedback. You can quickly and easily provide it by simply writing "Great job!" on the answer sheets or tests. For students who didn't perform well, a brief note such as "I'd love to talk with you at the end of class" can be especially reassuring. The key is to be proactive and maintain high standards, while requiring students to retain ownership of their success.

Managing Problem Situations

(From Philip C. Wankat, *The Effective, Efficient Professor: Teaching, Scholarship and Service,* published by Allyn & Bacon, Boston, MA. © 2002 by Pearson Education, Inc. Adapted by permission of the publisher.)

Cheating: Cheating is one behavior that should not be tolerated. Tolerating cheating tends to make it worse. Prevention of cheating is much more effective than trying to cure it once it has occurred. A professor can prevent cheating by:

- Creating rapport with students
- Gaining a reputation for giving fair tests
- Giving clear instructions and guidelines before, during, and after tests
- Educating students on the ethics of plagiarism
- Requiring periodic progress reports and outlines before a paper is due

Try to develop exams that are perceived as fair and secure by students. Often, the accusation that certain questions were tricky is valid as it relates to ambiguous language and trivial material. Ask your mentor or an experienced instructor to closely review the final draft of your first few exams for these factors.

(From David Royse, *Teaching Tips for College and University Instructors: A Practical Guide,* published by Allyn & Bacon, Boston, MA. © 2001 by Pearson Education, Inc. Adapted by permission of the publisher.)

Unmotivated students: There are numerous reasons why students may not be motivated. The "required course" scenario is a likely explanation—although politics in colonial America is your life's work, it is safe to assume that not everyone will share your enthusiasm. There are also personal reasons such as a death of a loved one or depression. Whenever you detect a pattern that you assume to be due to lack of motivation (e.g., missing classes, not handing assignments in on time, nonparticipation in class), arrange a time to have the student meet with you outside the classroom. Candidly express your concerns and then listen.

Tips for Thriving:

DISCIPLINE

One effective method for dealing with some discipline problems is to ask the class for feedback (Angelo & Cross, 1993). In a one-minute quiz, ask the students, "What can I do to help you learn?" Collate the responses and present them to the class. If behavior such as excessive talking appears in some responses (e.g., "Tell people to shut up"), this gives you the backing to ask students to be quiet. Use of properly channeled peer pressure is often effective in controlling undesired behavior.

Motivating students is part of the faculty members' job. To increase motivation, professors should show enthusiasm for the topic, use various media and methods to present material, use humor in the classroom, employ activities that encourage active learning, and give frequent, positive feedback.

(From Sharon Baiocco, & Jamie N. De Waters, *Successful College Teaching: Problem Solving Strategies of Distinguished Professors,* published by Allyn & Bacon, Boston, MA. © 1998 by Pearson Education, Inc. Adapted by permission of the publisher.)

Credibility problems: If you are an inexperienced instructor, you may have problems with students not taking you seriously. At the first class meeting, articulate clear rules of classroom decorum and conduct yourself with dignity and respect for students. Try to exude that you are in charge and are the "authority" and avoid trying to pose as the students' friend.

Improving Your Performance

(From Richard E. Lyons, Marcella L. Kysilka, & George E. Pawlas, *The Adjunct Professor's Guide to Success: Surviving and Thriving In The Classroom,* published by Allyn & Bacon, Boston, MA. © 1999 by Pearson Education, Inc. Adapted by permission of the publisher.)

Self-evaluation: The instructor who regularly engages in systematic self-evaluation will unquestionably derive greater reward from the formal methods of evaluation commonly employed by colleges and universities. One method for providing structure to an ongoing system of self-evaluation is to keep a journal of reflections on your teaching experiences. Regularly invest 15 or 20 introspective minutes following each class meeting to focus especially on the strategies and events in class that you feel could be improved. Committing your thoughts and emotions to writing enables you to develop more effective habits, build confidence in your teaching performance, and make more effective comparisons later. The following questions will help guide self-assessment:

How do I typically begin a class?

Where/How do I position myself in the class?

How do I move in the classroom?

Where are my eyes usually focused?

Do I facilitate students' visual processing of course material?

Do I change the speed, volume, energy, and tone of my voice?

How do I ask questions of students?

How often, and when, do I smile or laugh in class?

How do I react when students are inattentive?

How do I react when students disagree or challenge what I say?

How do I typically end a class?

Tips for Thriving:

VIDEO-RECORDING YOUR CLASS

In recent years, a wide range of professionals has markedly improved their job performance by employing video recorders in their preparation efforts. As an instructor, an effective method might be to ask your mentor or another colleague to tape a 10- to 15-minute mini-lesson, then to debrief it using the assessment questions above. Critiquing a videotaped session provides objectivity and is therefore more likely to effect change. Involving a colleague as an informal coach will enable you to gain from that person's experience and perspective and will reduce the chances of your engaging in self-depreciation.

References

Ailes, R. (1996). *You are the message: Getting what you want by being who you are.* New York: Doubleday.

Chickering, A. W., & Gamson, Z. F. (1987). "Seven principles for good practice in undergraduate education." *AAHE Bulletin,* 39, 3–7.

Michaelson, L. K. (1994). Team learning: Making a case for the small-group option. In K. W. Prichard & R. M. Sawyer (Eds.), *Handbook of college teaching.* Westport, CT: Greenwood Press.

Sorcinelli, M. D. (1991). Research findings on the seven principles. In A.W. Chickering & Z. Gamson (Eds.), "Applying the seven principles of good practice in undergraduate education." *New Directions for Teaching and Learning* 47. San Francisco: Jossey-Bass.

Teaching Tips for MyDietAnalysis

Teaching college students *about* nutrition is easy; having college students *learn and apply* nutrition is much more difficult! MyDietAnalysis (MDA) is a practical, "hands on" tool that can help ensure your students make the connection between textbook facts and real-life applications.

This primer, prepared by Carol Friesen, PhD, RD, from Ball State University, gives a brief introduction to MDA, providing an overview of how to integrate the program into your course (from navigating the actual MDA program, to providing discussion questions for classroom sessions, to incorporating MDA results into student homework assignments).

The Practical Aspects

Getting Started

Preparing the Food Record

- Prior to using *MyDietAnalysis*, instruct your students to write down everything they eat for as many days as you want to assign. Most teachers find a three-day food diary is adequate to capture the students' usual dietary intake without over-taxing them.
- To make the analysis as real as possible, encourage the students to select two typical weekdays and one weekend day, but to avoid holidays or days where they attended a special event such as a state fair or an "open house."
- For the results of the diet analysis to be accurate, you will probably have to teach the students to identify *how much* of each food they eat. Most teachers do this by demonstrating standard serving sizes using a variety of common household items (e.g., 3 ounces of meat = a deck of cards; 1/2 cup of a vegetable or fruit = a tennis ball). Lists of these common serving sizes are found in your textbook. I ask for two volunteers (one male, one female) to come to the front of the room to pour out the amount of breakfast cereal they typically eat and then I both weigh and measure the amount of cereal. Rarely does the amount equal the standard serving of 1 ounce or 1 cup.
- Now would be a good time to ask your students to bring at least one food label to class. Show your students how to identify the number of servings in each unit of food. Point out how they can use the number of servings, and serving size per unit, to help them identify how much they ate—whether in grams or ounces or cups.
- Remind your students to be *very specific* when they record WHAT they ate (e.g., write down "Cheerios," not "cereal"; fat-free milk, not "milk"; 2 ounces of ham, 2 slices whole wheat bread, 1 tsp mayonnaise, NOT "a sandwich").
- Instruct the students to record HOW MUCH they ate, encouraging them to use labels as often as possible to estimate the serving size in ounces or cups. Remind your students the more accurate THEY are, the more accurate the RESULTS will be!

Using MyDietAnalysis

- Once the students have their food lists, they are ready to enter the data into MyDietAnalysis. They do this by going to CourseCompass (http://course compass.com), selecting your nutrition course, and clicking on MyDietAnalysis (fourth red button on the left). This will direct you to a screen with a delicious looking green apple.
- Click on "Enter MyDietAnalysis" – the button in the middle of the green apple.
- The students will now enter their **PROFILE INFORMATION**. They will need to provide their birthdate, height, weight, gender, activity level (click on the down arrow to choose from the selection). NOTE: It is at this point students can indicate if they want to LOSE or GAIN WEIGHT. **If the student wants to lose weight, they must enter -0.5 or -1.0 lbs per week (i.e., MINUS)**. If you want to GAIN weight, just put down 1 or 2. Overweight students should calculate their energy and nutrient needs based on their desirable, not actual, weight.
- If you would prefer, the students can complete a 24-hour activity profile to get a more accurate estimate of their usual activity; most, however, find it easier just to assess their life and select from the drop-down options (e.g., from 'sedentary' to 'extremely active').
- Once this information is entered, the student's individual DRI goals will be calculated.
- Next, it is time to enter the foods. The students will click on the **INTAKE** tab on the top of the page (second tab from the left; next to PROFILE tab). Specifically, the program asks each student to:
  a. Start with Day 1. Type in the food you ate. Be careful of spelling. If you aren't a good speller, or if you can't find a food, try using the asterisk trick – for example, if you ate cantaloupe, type cant* and a listing of all the foods that start with 'cant' will pop up. If you can't find a food the first time, try again! Try using the brand name, (e.g., McD* for McDonald's), the food type (e.g., hamb* for hamburger, dress* for salad dressing), or a food category (e.g., 'candy' or 'salad').
  b. Click on the food. Next, select the MEAL (this is not essential) and the AMOUNT and MEASURE of each food (this IS essential!). For example, let's say you put 1/2 cup of fat-free milk on cereal. Type "MILK" – select "FAT FREE MILK with VITAMINS A and D," click "BREAKFAST," type "4" and then click "OUNCES" (for 4 ounces) *or* type "0.5" and then click "CUP" for 1/2 cup. When done, click ENTER to include the food in your analysis.
  c. Continue to add all the foods eaten throughout the day. Any repeat foods become easy to select because they are in the drop down box; they will show up each time you start to type that food's name.
  d. When you are done with Day 1, click the tab (left-hand side of screen) that says Day 2. Repeat the process, including up to seven days of food.

MyDietAnalysis Output

Finally, it is time to get the output! Encourage your students to keep these printouts in a safe place (I recommend a plastic sleeve) and to bring the printouts to class every day.

- Click on the **REPORT** tab. Scroll to the bottom. Select **ALL DAILY REPORTS**. This will provide a comprehensive printout of each day PLUS the average nutrient intake over all the days you entered.

- On average, you will end up with about 10–15 pages of reports (it depends how much you eat!). Be prepared with enough paper and ink!
- I always have the students hand in their 3-day printouts very early in the semester. I give them "all or nothing" points for this part of the assignment (e.g., 5 points for turning it in by the deadline). I look over the printouts to identify any errors—then I hand it back to the students so they can make any necessary corrections before they use it in any analysis. Typical errors include students who say they drank 1 gallon of milk (rather than 1 cup), or ate 1 pizza pie (rather than 1 piece of pizza), or had 10 packages of 10-piece chicken nuggets (rather than one 10-piece package of nuggets), or drank 1 cup powdered lemonade (rather than 1 cup lemonade made from powder!), or ate 1 loaf of bread rather than 1 slice. This quality check is very important . . . their results are meaningless if what is analyzed doesn't represent the truth.
- A few tips to speed up the checking process—I typically turn immediately to the printout that lists total calories consumed and lists the caloric contribution of each food. When I see a caloric level that is inappropriate (i.e., too low or too high), it is a red flag. I scrutinize the list of foods to identify which one is the culprit and I circle that food for the student to see.

In the Classroom

Using the MyDiet Analysis Results to Enhance Classroom Learning

I am convinced that, after having taught nutrition at the college level for over 20 years, integrating the results of a students diet analysis is the most effective way to translate facts into "Aha! I get it!" moments! Let me share with you a few examples of how I integrate the diet analysis into my nutrition teaching.

Getting Ready

- Over time, I have found it convenient to create what I call a "Summary Sheet," a two-column single-page sheet onto which the students transfer key information needed throughout the class and during the written diet analysis assignment. I break the summary sheet into "Energy", "Carbohydrate," "Protein," "Lipids," and "Vitamins/Minerals" sections. The students abstract the DRI, the amount consumed, the percent consumed, etc. from their printouts onto the summary sheet. Using the summary sheet saves a significant amount of time when I ask questions in class as the students don't have to dig through the reports to find the correct information.
- If you make a summary sheet, make sure the students provide the correct information; when you ask for the RDA for protein, make sure they give you the RDA. When you ask for percent of calories from CHO, make sure they give you percent of calories from CHO, not percent of recommended grams of CHO consumed.
- I assign the summary sheet AFTER the students have received their corrected 3-day diet analysis printouts. That way you know the information they are transferring from the diet analysis forms to the nutrient summary sheet is accurate. I do require the students to hand in both the nutrient summary sheet AND their 3-day analysis printouts just so I can make sure they are transferring the right numbers. A little extra time at the beginning of the semester saves a lot of headaches when the written diet analysis assignment is due.

Food Guide Pyramid

- Having the students memorize the number of recommended servings of foods from each food group is pointless, particularly with the current MyPyramid version that has 12 combinations based on age and gender and that focuses on ounces and cups rather than on servings. The MyPyramid graph indicates how many ounces and cups are recommended for each student and how many (or how few) servings were consumed by the students over the three days.
- By show of hands, ask the class how many are low in each of the various groups. Ask how — based on their crazy lifestyles the foods available to them, and their likes and dislikes — they can increase the number of servings to meet the recommendations. Encourage the students to select one food group in which they are particularly low to see if they can make changes over the coming week. Don't forget to follow up! Ask HOW they were able to make changes.
- Later in the course, while you are covering the vitamins and minerals, return to the MyPyramid section of the diet analysis. Ask the students to closely examine their vitamin A, C, potassium and folic acid consumption in comparison to their fruit and vegetable consumption. Is there any relationship? How about between their calcium and vitamin D intake and their milk and dairy consumption? Between their iron and B_{12} intake and their protein intake? Remind the students that, if they apply the concepts of variety and moderation, they won't *have* to complete the time-consuming diet analysis if they ate the MyPyramid way!

Carbohydrates

- You will teach your students that, to be healthy, it is recommended that they consume between 45–65% of their calories from carbohydrate. It's a great fact . . . but does it *really* mean? Have their students pull out their MyDietAnalysis results! Have them locate the section that lists the percent of calories from macronutrients. Did they meet the requirement? Were they high? Low?
- Have the students cross-reference the percent of calories they consumed with the number of ounces from the Bread and Cereal group. Is there a relationship?
- Look at the grams of sugar consumed. It is recommended that adults consume no more than 40–50 grams of sugar per day (approximately 10 teaspoons). Ask the students how many grams they consumed. What percent of the recommended amount did they consume? What percent of their total calories came from sugar? It is also recommended that no more than 10% of one's calories come from refined sugar.
- Ask the class if someone has a bottle of soda with them. Have them look at the label and tell you how many grams of sugar there are per serving. Ask them how many ounces is in the bottle. How many *servings* are in the bottle? How much sugar are they consuming if they drank the entire bottle? Students often don't realize a 20 ounce bottle of soda is more than one serving. Most students perceive a 'serving' as the amount they eat.
- I always demonstrate how much sugar is in various foods by measuring sugar, teaspoon by teaspoon (or directly onto a gram scale), into a clear class bowl. For example, I ask the students to tell me "STOP" when they think I have measured the amount of sugar in a 20 ounce bottle of soda. It just about makes the students gag!
- Ask a volunteer to come to the front of the room to measure out how much sugar they consumed, on average, over the three days. Then take that amount

and multiply it by seven to indicate how much sugar they consume in one week. It is an eye opening experience.

- Next, take a look at the fiber content of the student's diet. Ask the students, by show of hands, how many consumed 100% of their recommended amount of total fiber. Encourage the student to cross-check their fiber intake with their total number of ounces/cups of fruits, vegetables, and whole grains they consumed. Is there a relationship?
- Identify a student who has consumed the most fiber in the class (hopefully you have validated their results by checking their printouts!). Make a table with the headings "Fiber, gm", "Fruits," "Vegetables," and "Grains." Fill in the chart with the number of these food groups they consumed. Repeat this for the person who consumed the least amount of fiber. Can you see the relationship between the two?? Did anyone make 'half their grains whole'? Find someone who ate chili or refried beans or baked beans. How did that impact their fiber intake?

Fat/Lipids

- MyDietAnalysis really helps the students understand many of the complex issues associated with lipids. Have the students identify how many total grams of fat they consumed and what percent of their calories came from fat. Did they meet the recommended 15–35% of calories from fat?
- Next, we look at the types of fat the students consumed. It is helpful to have a volunteer name a food they consumed (e.g., lasagna) and then, using the printout that lists the sources of nutrients from each food, have them tell how much total fat there was in the food, and how much of the total fat was saturated, monounsaturated, and polyunsaturated. Most students think foods are "all or nothing" when it comes to types of fat (e.g., either all saturated or all monounsaturated). This helps them understand foods contain a mixture of types of fat.
- Examine the saturated fat content of a volunteer's diet. Identify the percent of the fat calories that came from saturated fat. Were more than one-third of their fat calories saturated? If so, what types of foods contributed saturated fat to the diet? Calculate the percent of total calories from saturated fat (i.e., multiply grams of saturated fat by 9 kcals/gram and divide that product by the total calories consumed). Did they meet the current recommendation of less than seven percent of calories from saturated fat?
- Next examine the monounsaturated and polyunsaturated content of the diet. Did they eat more grams of monounsaturated fat and polyunsaturated fat when compared to grams of saturated fat? Look at the P:S ratio on the MyDietAnalysis printout. Discuss ways they could improve their fat intake and type. What were good sources of monounsaturated fat in the students' diets?
- Have the students examine their cholesterol intake. Memorizing "less than 300 milligrams per day" is one thing; realizing they are eating 440 mg per day is another! All of a sudden, the goal numbers become more real; they have meaning. In class discussion, we talk about specific dietary changes they could make to meet the recommended fat guidelines. We also discuss how most students are afraid to eat eggs. By show of hands, ask how many students' diets met the recommended cholesterol intake. From my experience, most college students are well below the recommended 300 mg or less of cholesterol per day. I encourage the students not to avoid eggs; they are an inexpensive, quick to prepare, high quality protein food that has 'staying power' in the refrigerator. In essence, the egg could be the student's favorite fast food (next to fruits and vegetables, of course!).

Protein

- After discussing the DRI for protein (0.8 gm/kg for adults), have the students examine their protein DRI. Can they see how it was calculated using the formula and their weight? If they don't believe you, have them repeat step one of the MyDietAnalysis, but this time pretending they weighed 100 pounds more than they currently do. See how the protein DRI has increased?
- Ask how many grams of protein the students consumed, on average. What percent of their calories came from protein? How does this compare to the recommended level (10–35% pf calories). What percent of their DRI did they consume? Did they eat more than 200% of their DRI? If so, their liver (deamination) and their pocket book (protein foods are expensive compared to other energy foods) are both paying a high price for this energy-yielding nutrient. Have the students discuss what substitutions they could make in their diets so they get the energy they need from carbohydrate rather than from protein.
- Do you have any vegans in your class? Lacto-ovo vegetarians? Were they able to consume adequate protein compared to meat eaters?
- The protein recommendation is often controversial among the athletes in your nutrition class. Be prepared! Remind the students that current science *does* recommend athletes consume up to 2.0 grams of protein per kilogram (compared to 0.8 grams per kilogram for non-athletes). Students who engage in strenuous physical activity should be encouraged to re-calculate their DRI for protein and hand-calculate their percent DRI consumed.

Vitamins and Minerals

- By show of hands, ask how many were deficient in a certain vitamin or mineral (I use < 75% DRI as my cut-off point for deficient). The students begin to see that a lot of them have the same deficiencies that need to be addressed; they are able to support one another as they seek alternate nutritious foods. Try making a bar graph indicating how many students are deficient in each vitamin or mineral. Then ask students who were not deficient in each vitamin or mineral to report what foods they consumed that were good nutrient sources.
- This is also a good time to reinforce the material from the beginning of the course where you tried to explain how the DRIs were established and, specifically, why individuals don't *have* to consume 100% of the DRI to avoid a nutrient deficiency. Specifically, I ask the students whether or not they think eating less than 100% of the DRI over the three days for any nutrient is a cause for concern. They must defend their answers!
- In the written portion of the diet analysis assignment, I require the students to list at least three food sources *they would enjoy eating* that would provide the vitamins and minerals lacking in their diets. Light-heartedly, I tell them if "liver" is included in the list, they will be invited to my house for a liver and onion dinner to prove they like it!
- Once again, the vitamins/minerals unit is a great time to stress the relationship between the MISSING vitamins and minerals in their diet and the DEFICIENT FOOD GROUPS in their diet.

Summary

Simply put, I cannot imagine teaching a nutrition class without using a comprehensive diet analysis throughout the entire semester! This tool reinforces the sometimes-confusing dietary recommendations, especially for the mathematically challenged. I urge all nutrition teachers to integrate the MyDietAnalysis into lectures as often as possible, so the students can truly begin to understand that what they eat makes a difference to their health.

Tips for Using MyNutritionLab

The MyNutritionLab is a course management system that can be used to manage an online class or as a complement to any nutrition course. Materials can be customized to provide your students with preloaded course materials or with course contents you load for them.

MyNutritionLab (MNL) offers premium online content, including textbook quizzes, ABC News Lecture Launcher video clips, animations and activities, and much more. Once students are logged into the MNL course site, they are also set up in a CourseCompass gradebook which will automatically record all scores and assignments completed through MNL.

This primer gives a brief introduction to MNL, providing an overview of how to integrate these resources into your course (from navigating the actual program to providing assignments for classroom sessions) to using MNL to enhance lecture content and to assign student homework. Sample assignments are also included here to illustrate ways MNL will enhance your course and increase student involvement. This primer is modified from the original created by Barbara Hewitt, M.S., from Diablo Valley College.

The Practical Aspects

MNL is hosted by CourseCompass. After creating your CourseCompass log in you will need to log in again to customize your course. When you log in, it opens to the My CourseCompass page. CourseCompass is organized by four tabs that appear at the top of the right of the page: My CourseCompass, Courses, Services, and Research Navigator™. Your course will appear on the My CourseCompass page. For full instructions on how to set up a CourseCompass course and provide access to students, click the Getting Started with CourseCompass link on the far right side of your My CourseCompass page.

After registering, you can begin to tailor the content to meet your needs. Most of the set up and customization is initiated from the Control Panel, a link to which appears on the bottom of the left-hand navigation bar. These Control Panel items are visible to you but not your students.

Working with the Control Panel

Content Areas

The content area of the control panel includes the Course Information, Study Tools, Chapter Contents, Assignments, and Instructor Tools sections. In course information, you will find all software requirements to run MNL and downloads if needed. This is an excellent place to load in your syllabus and a personal biography or vitae.

Study Tools (preloaded content)

Items in this section are preloaded animations, Research Navigator™, eBook, eThemes of the *New York Times* articles, Web links, quizzes, glossary, and flashcards.

The section on eThemes is a valuable resource offering a collection of 30 contemporary articles from the *New York Times*. The articles are current and related to each chapter. These are useful for students to summarize for extra credit or to outline prior to a lecture. Research

Navigator™ is a helpful tool for students, allowing them access to scholarly journals and other valuable Internet nutrition resource sites.

Instructors can choose to use all or some of these resources by simply clicking the copy, modify, or remove icons throughout MNL control panel.

Chapter Contents (preloaded content)

The items loaded into Chapter Contents include text-based resources and more, including the full chapter of the eBook, animations, ABC News Lecture Launcher Videos, practice quizzes, Nutrition Debate activities, chapter objectives, flashcards, answers to the Nutri-Case case studies, and answers to the Find the Quack features. These items can be modified or removed for use in your class or assigned for homework. Chapter practice quizzes and Nutrition Debate activities are particularly useful to use as homework assignments to reinforce chapter comprehension. The ABC News video clips that are available here are excellent tools to introduce your topics in lecture.

Assignments and External Links (some preloaded content)

The ability to post assignments and external links allows instructors to load personal course assignment instructions and links to other areas on the Internet. A nice use for this area is to load any assignment instruction sheets, review sheets, and/or your PowerPoint lectures for student viewing. An example of how to use both of these would be to load your PowerPoint lecture into the course as or link to it as an external link and include an assignment to complete after viewing the PowerPoint lecture. For example, after students view the PowerPoint ask them to answer a worksheet (loaded into assignment section) with questions about the content that was just covered. This can be printed out and brought to class or sent directly to your email for grading or put in the digital drop box for your viewing later. MNL has seven preloaded assignments for use with MyDietAnalysis. These assignments are extremely helpful in showing students how to analyze diet analysis reports.

Course Tools

This area of MNL is an area for personalizing your content and creating a course calendar. Each section may or may not be made available to your students to use for email, handing in assignments (digital drop box), or obtaining staff information. If you use MNL as a stand-alone course, this area works well for classroom management. When MNL is purely a complement to your lecture classes, you may choose to remove many of these options. It has been my experience that the non-online students already feel bombarded with materials in class and providing too many outside materials may be overwhelming. Sometimes providing only the materials distributed in class as required materials works the best. Be careful not to overload your MNL with unnecessary items that might distract students from the required content and assignments for your course. The area I use most is Send Email, sending emails to students to remind them of tests, assignments or class cancellations.

Announcements

The Announcement area is another area I use often and set as my opening page. As described on page 116, I change it weekly and update all assignment information, class lecture content and test information. This is where I describe the weekly assignments and readings due and any other announcements regarding class.

Discussion Board

The Discussion Board is particularly useful for bringing students together to discuss amongst themselves (either anonymously or by name) controversial issues or topics. A forum can be posted for students to write about and reply to other students with comments. This is valuable to use when a class discussion isn't finished or needs more exploration. The discussion responses can be organized alphabetically and printed out for grading at any time. They can also be stored as an archive, for viewing at a later date.

Course Options

The Manage Course Menu and Manage Tools areas are found in this section. This is where you choose which tool-bar icons you will make available to your students and how you will display them. Remember, try not to overload students and to only post the items you will be using in your course, i.e., don't make the digital drop box available if you want your students to hand in assignments in class. I use this area to add any other icon or materials to the course. For example, this is where I load the PowerPoint lectures I use in class so students can refer to them to study for tests or obtain lecture notes if they missed class. I name this tool Lecture Notes, and place it in the tool area of CourseCompass as a separate icon.

User Management

This section is helpful to use to enhance group project work and provide necessary group project materials for all students to access and/or store their work for group members to view or to work together.

Assessment

An excellent tool for instructors' use in administering tests, surveying students, and storing grades, MNL automatically posts grades from quizzes and other assessments, which save instructors a lot of grading time. TestGen is the test making program MNL uses. I use this to create practice tests or timed tests.

Help

This area is for instructors to access technical support and CourseCompass help.

MyNutritionLab in the Classroom

Using MNL to Enhance Classroom Learning

After navigating the Control Panel, you can now plan some ways to use this in your class. I use MNL both as a classroom supplement and as a stand-alone online class for students to use to access class materials and complete assignments.

One of the most useful tools on MNL are the video lecture launchers. Gone are the days of VCR and VHS or DVD. Now, you can access these excellent videos from your laptop and then easily open your PowerPoint slides to start the lecture. The answers to the Nutri-Cases are also nice lecture introductions to open a discussion of how this chapter relates to students lives.

Another useful way to use MNL in class is to build flashcards to close your lecture content at the end. Have students work in pairs to find the definition of the term and raise their hand if they know the answer. If they are right, I give them 1 extra credit point. Sometimes, I show the definition card and have them try to find the term instead. The Flashcard feature is found under Study Tools.

The video lecture launchers, the case studies and the flashcards are three ways MNL can enhance student involvement and learning in the classroom. Occasionally, I will assign the practice quizzes to complete in class or as homework.

MyNutritionLab Online Course

Setting up an online class takes time, particularly in the nutrition sciences, as course materials need to be updated frequently and the assignments need to reflect the new content. Having said this, the preloaded content of MNL, makes this task somewhat easier. The challenge is to choose materials which equate to the required time per unit at your school and to offer an online class experience that provides some interaction and teacher involvement. For example, for a 3 semester unit class, the estimated hours of work for a student is 3 in-class hours/week and approximately 2–3 study hours outside of class. Therefore, when a student is taking your class online, they need to spend 5–6 hours/week working on the assignments and readings for this class.

For classroom management, I also make my online class correspond closely to my face-to-face class, so students can use them interchangeably and course planning is easier when we are all doing the same assignments. Online teaching demands a new pedagogy from instructors. It is harder to interact with the class and to integrate your teaching styles into the online format. In some ways, online teaching allows for more individual teaching (through email) and thus allows for a more personalized experience; yet, students do not get to work closely with each other as they do in a classroom setting. There are pros and cons to online classes and as instructors I believe we are still trying to determine the most effective ways to provide the best experience online. Here are some suggestions to make the course as productive as possible.

Orientation

To best allow students to succeed in an online class, I require an introductory face-to–face 2-hour orientation. Together we enroll in CourseCompass, browse the site, and download the syllabus, assignments and calendar. Students tend to have issues with access codes and/or plug-ins or system requirements with their home computers, so doing this orientation is crucial. I suggest that students set up a "virtual" classroom at home with their computer and a bulletin board with the syllabus, the assignments, the discussion items, calendar and the quizzes for each chapter. This way, each week they can refer to a hard copy of the discussion, assignments or quizzes. They can work on them at other times throughout the day and answer them first on paper before submitting them for grading. I do not require timed tests online because I still require students to come on campus for three proctored tests with me.

During orientation, I run a class exercise for students to get to know each other and begin to relate as a class and online. For example, have them respond to a discussion item about "What is Nutrition?" and reply to someone else's definition; we then discuss these in class. Students can then see who everyone is and begin to feel more comfortable navigating the site and interacting with each other online.

Weekly Announcements

This section is what I use for my opening page. Students see these when the open their MNL. Each week I post the required class assignments, readings and due dates. For example:

Week of 10/29/08

1. Please read Chapter 1 and answer the four multiple choice quizzes and Nutrition Debate assignment, due Friday at 2 pm. Nutrition Debate assignments need to be submitted to the drop box. Quizzes are graded and recorded automatically when you hit "submit"
2. Diet Analysis Assessment assignment is also due next week, remember to review the assignment instructions under the assignment section. You should be working on this.
3. Discussion item is also posted and due on Friday by 2 pm.

Under Options in the Announcement Modification section, I choose to always show all announcements throughout the semester so students can see the last week's assignments as well.

Preloaded Tests

Each week students will take the preloaded tests for at least one chapter (sometimes two). These tests are automatically graded and organized in your gradebook section in MNL. I like to know my students are reading the text and understand the terms and concepts. Students can print these out and work on them in hard copy before submitting them online. Therefore, they are open book tests. Each test is answered then submitted and the correct answers can be viewed. Under the Test Options section, I set the tests so that they can only take them once. The students can view the tests, but once they take the test, they are done. I give 100 semester points for completing all chapter tests. They must have of at least 70% correct to get credit. The tests are due weekly and are emailed directly to me. They must be saved on the students desktop first. You can also load a TestGen test, which can be scored and submitted directly to the gradebook.

Discussion

Each week students are required to respond and reply (to at least on other person) to a discussion topic related to the weekly content. I post all discussion items at the beginning of the semester, so students can print these out and think about them from a hard copy before replying. Sometimes, these discussions require outside research. For example, I ask students to research their local food bank and describe the services they offer. I also require a grocery store field trip with a label viewing assignment. There are some good questions for discussion and reflection found in the beginning of each chapter. Other sample discussion forums include:

1. What are the benefits and drawbacks of a low-carbohydrate, high-protein diet? What if someone you know is at risk for cardiovascular disease and they want to try a high-protein diet to lose weight? Would you recommend that they do so or not? Why?
2. Discuss three ideas to curb the rising rates of childhood obesity.
3. Vitamin and mineral supplements are used widely. Discuss two supplements you have used or been interested in using and why that may or may not be a good idea.

Allowing anonymous posting on discussion items may allow for more sharing of information here. Although, with this option, instructors do not know which students have participated. I have used this anonymous posting option for sensitive issues, and they have lead to some very intimate discussions.

Assignments

I require seven assignments outside of the text (approximately one every other week). Some of these can be done in pairs, most are done alone. For a nutrition research assignment, students can use the Research Navigator tool to find five sources to use to research information on a nutrition issue of their choice. There are also seven preloaded diet analysis assignments in this section on MNL.

Assignment groups can be formed by using the Manage Groups section of the Control Panel. I set up group discussion boards, and group sharing through this section, and later I can see what work was done by whom.

Other possible assignments are: personal nutrition review, assessing nutrition information, a fitness plan, a diet analysis (using MyDietAnalysis), and research on a nutrition supplement of their choice. Instructions for assignment formats, requirements and submission are all loaded into the assignment section.

Assignment Example: Assessing nutrition information using e-Themes of the Times

Accessing and assessing accurate nutrition information is a course objective in many nutrition courses. One assignment to explore nutrition information resources is to ask students to read a *NY Times* article from the e-Themes in the Study Tools section. Explain that the *NY Times* article is a secondary source and ask students to find three other sources mentioned in the article and locate them. Then ask them to distinguish between a primary, secondary, and tertiary source.

You can post a document in the Assignment section with the assignment instructions and a worksheet to be answered and emailed directly to you or placed in the Drop Box. Some question you can have students answer are:

1. Why would you choose a newspaper article to access nutrition information?
2. Describe what you learned from the other sources you found. How does it differ from what you read in the newspaper article?
3. What are the differences between a primary, secondary, and tertiary sources?
4. What is the "Web" good for?
5. What is the difference between a .org and a .com site?

Proctored Tests

I do not use the timed TestGen tests preloaded in MNL but prefer to require students take two midterms and a final with me. During the exams, students can also discuss problems, assignments, or nutrition issues that the course brought up for them. Through the 3 years I have been teaching online, I believe these students perform as well or better than my face-to-face students on tests. They are required to read the text and become more disciplined with their study habits. Some students do not succeed in an online class, but the many who do have disciplined themselves to "show up" at their virtual classroom and do their work.

Sample Syllabi

Sample Syllabus for Introduction to Nutrition: 12-week Course

Course: Biology 370 – Principles of Nutrition. MTh 3:30 – 4:45 pm

Faculty:

Office: **Phone:** **e-mail:**

Office Hours: Mon. 2:00–3:00 p.m., Tues. 3:00–5:00 p.m., and Wed. 3:00–5:00 p.m.

Other hours by appointment.

Course Text:

Nutrition: An Applied Approach, 2e. 2009, Thompson and Manore

Course Description: Development of an understanding of normal adult nutrition based on learning the chemical and physiological processes of nutrient selection, digestion, absorption, and metabolism. Selected nutritionally influenced diseases will also be discussed with respect to cause and/or management. 3 quarter units.

Goals: Upon completion of lecture and reading assignments, the student will be able to:

1. Describe the role of nutrients and ways nutrition affects adult human health.
2. Describe the food groups, food labels, and Dietary Guidelines and the research processes leading to these guidelines.
3. Describe the chemical and physiological processes of nutrient selection, digestion, absorption, transportation, and metabolism.
4. Describe the energy balance and body weight, and conditions that affect them.
5. Describe the role of nutrition in maintaining a healthy body.
6. Identify and describe eating disorders that can be detrimental to human health.
7. Describe and identify factors which can cause diseases such as obesity, cardiovascular disease, diabetes, hypertension, and cancer.

Class Hours:

Lecture: MTh 3:30 - 4:45 am. Reading assignments are listed. The reading and lecture complement each other. Not every detail can be covered in lecture; however, you will be responsible for the material in the chapters assigned. **Plan on reading before each lecture, and be able to participate in class discussions**. You may use an audio recording device in class if that helps, but please let me know about this in writing.

Evaluation

Exam I	**100 pts**
Exam II	**100 pts**
Diet Analysis	**50 pts**
Class Activities	**50 pts**
Final	**100 pts**
Total Points	**400 pts**

See the University Catalog for information concerning plagiarism and academic dishonesty. Cheating is totally unacceptable, and will be reported.

Lecture Exams: Exams may be in multiple choice, matching, fill-in-the-blanks, and true false format. The final can include material from previous exams, but will mainly include material presented after the last exam.

Diet Analysis: Handouts will be given in class after the first week of lectures. This project must be submitted on time.

Class Activities: These can include in class exercises, assignments, and class discussions. If you miss this *for any reason*, there is ***NO make up*** assignment, and you will receive a ZERO for that day.

Grading Policy

100%–94 = A	82–80 = B-	69–67 = D+
92–90 = A-	79–77 = C+	66–63 = D
89–87 = B+	76–73 = C	62–60 = D-
86–83 = B	72–70 = C-	59–0 = F

Class Policies

Attendance Policy—It is important to show up to class since you and I have paid the tuition fees. It is up to you to decide, since the exams may contain some material discussed in class that may not necessarily be in your book, as well as for class activities. You snooze, you lose.

Make-up Exam Policy—Missed exams due to illness or other justified reasons may be made up. If you know in advance that you must miss an exam, see me and bring *documentation* to support your anticipated absence. If you miss an exam unexpectedly because of last-minute illness or an accident contact me when you return to campus (or by phone if you will be away for some time) with *documentation* of your situation. **The decision remains with the instructor. There is no make-up for the final**.

Special Needs—If you have special needs because of learning or other kinds of disabilities, please feel free to come and discuss this with me. I am available for *individual consultation* regarding any aspect of the course. If you have unanswered questions or concerns, or are in serious academic trouble, see me before it is too late! Make an appointment; come during office hours, phone, or e-mail a message.

Tentative Lecture Schedule

Date	Topic	Chapter
Mar 27	The Role of Nutrition in Our Health	1
Mar 30	Designing a Healthful Diet	2
April 3	The Human Body: Are we really what we eat?	3
	Begin diet log/diary for three weeks	
April 6	Carbohydrates: Bountiful Sources of Energy and Nutrients	4
April 10	Fat: An Essential Energy Supplying Nutrient	5
	Week 1 of food diary due.	
April 13	Proteins: Crucial Components of All Body Tissues	6
April 17	Follow-up Day	
April 20	**Exam I**	
	Week 2 of food diary due.	
April 24	Nutrients involved in Fluid and Electrolyte Balance	7
April 27	Nutrients involved in Antioxidant Function	8
May 1	Nutrients involved in Bone Health	9
	Week 3 of food diary due.	
May 4	Nutrients involved in Energy Metabolism and Blood Health	10
May 8	Achieving and Maintaining a Healthful Body Weight	11
May 11	Follow-up Day	
May 15	**Exam II**	
May 18	Nutrition and Physical Activity	12
	Diet Analysis Due.	
May 22	Nutrition and Physical Activity (Continued)	
May 25	Disordered Eating	13
May 29	Holiday (Memorial Day) No Classes	
June 1	Food Safety and Technology	14
June 5	Nutrition through the Lifecycle: Pregnancy and the first year Chapter 16 Assigned Reading	15

Final Exam: TBA.

Sample Syllabus for Introduction to Nutrition: 16-week Course

NTR 100 - INTRODUCTORY NUTRITION (3)

SPRING SEMESTER, 2007

Lecture: MW, 1:25-2:15 p.m.; WLS M309

Discussion Sections:

Friday:	8:00-8:50	414 JHB	10:10-11:00	414 JHB	12:20-1:10	413 JHB
	9:05-9:55	414 JHB	11:15-12:05	414 JHB	1:25-2:15	414 JHB (6)

Note: JHB is Jessie Harris Bldg.

A. Personal Information:

Instructor:

Office:

Telephone:

Office Hours: M, W—9:00–10:00 a.m. or by appointment

Email:

Teaching Assistants:

NOTE: Messages can be left in faculty and teaching assistant's departmental mail boxes in 229 JHB.

PREREQUISITES: None

B. Course Description:

Nutritional concepts; current consumer issues in nutrition; nutritional needs through life cycle; international nutrition concerns and/or issues. A student who has received credit for NTR 300 may not receive credit for this course.

C. Objectives:

To introduce the student to basic nutrition information and how the application of this information may contribute to good health.

Student Objectives:

At the conclusion of this class, students will be expected to:

1. Understand basic nutrition concepts as they apply to normal nutrition.
2. Recognize the contribution of foods and their nutrients to good health throughout the lifespan.
3. Analyze his/her own personal dietary habits and be motivated to improve them, if necessary.
4. Understand the contribution of diet to common health problems in the U.S. and the world.
5. Use basic nutrition knowledge to analyze current nutrition fads and fallacies.

D. Course Requirements:

1. *Examination Policy:*

Students are expected to take four equally weighted tests and one final exam. Tests will be multiple choice and are scheduled on the course calendar. **There are no make-up exams**. The lowest score of the four hourly examinations will be dropped. Examination results will not be given over the phone under any circumstances. Grades will be posted in a display case two school days after each examination. Display case is located at the East end of the ground floor of Jessie Harris Building adjacent to Room 16. Examination results will also be posted on the web.

2. *Academic Honesty Statement:*

Student Academic Conduct from the latest **HILLTOPICS** will be followed.

Exclusion from the University or any lesser penalty may result from any of the following misconducts;

#1 from **"Standards of Conduct"**

Academic cheating or plagiarism,

#7 from **"Standards of Conduct"**

Obstruction or disruption of teaching, research, administration, disiplanary procedings, or other University activities, including public service functions, or of any authorized activities on University premises.

3. *Class Attendance:*

Class attendance is strongly encouraged as there is a positive correlation between class attendance and grades. Frequently material that is not in your readings is presented in class. Attendance in discussion is mandatory. Students are allowed one unexcused absence throughout the semester. Total discussion grade will decrease 4% for each additional absence.

4. *Textbook:*

Thompson/Manore. Nutrition: An Applied Approach, 2nd edition. 2009. Pearson.

5. *Assignments:*

Reading assignments from the text are listed on the course calendar. Additional assignments will be made in class. No late assignments will be accepted without permission of your Teaching Assistant.

6. *Teaching Techniques:*

Lectures with audio-visual materials will be held in 416 Dougherty Building with some discussion. Smaller group in-class discussion sessions will meet to focus on specific topics with the teaching assistants in Jessie Harris Building.

7. *Criteria for Evaluation of Student Performance:*

a. There will be 4 equally weighted tests which will account for 50% of the course grade. (The lowest score will be dropped).

b. Discussion group assignments and attendance will account for 25% of the course grade.

c. A comprehensive final exam will account for 25% of the course grade.

8. *Grading Scale:*

   Final letter grades will be assigned as follows:

   A = 90.0 – 100%

   B+ = 87.0 – 89.9%

   B = 80.0 – 86.9%

   C+ = 77.0 – 79.9%

   C = 70.0 – 76.9%

   D = 60.0 – 69.9% F = < 60%

9. *Late Assignments:*

   No late projects will be accepted without TA permission and a 10% per day penalty.

10. *Snow Day Policy:*

    The general UTK policy for snow days is in effect. The University is open unless you hear the closure announced on radio/TV. However, if an exam is scheduled on a day on which we have snow, the exam will be postponed until the next class day to accommodate off-campus transportation problems.

11. *Feedback Policy:*

    Two school days after each of the (4) one hour examinations, grades will be posted in a glass case in the hallway outside room 16 Jessie Harris Building (East end, basement). The examination with answers will also be posted at this time. The examination and answers will remain posted until the next examination is given. For example; exam 1 will be posted 48 hours after it is given until the day Exam 2 is given. Exam 1 will not be retrievable after Exam 2 is given. This is the policy for all 4 hourly examinations.

12. Students who have a disability that require accommodation(s) should make an appointment with the Office of Disability Services to discuss their specific needs as well as schedule an appointment with me during office hours.

TENTATIVE COURSE CALENDAR NTR 100

Date	Lecture Topic	Text Chapter	Discussion Topic	Text Pages
1/10 W	Nutrition and Health	1		
1/12 F			Food Guide Pyramid	51–67
1/15 M	**HOLIDAY (MLK Day)**			
1/17 W	Designing a Healthful Diet	2		
1/19 F			Reading Labels	40–48
1/22 M	Digestion and Absorption	3		
1/24 W	Digestion and Absorption	3		
1/26 F			Alcohol	160–169
1/29 M	**EXAMINATION 1**	**1–3**		
1/31 W	Carbohydrate	4		
2/2 F			Diabetes	146–151
2/5 M	Carbohydrate	4		
2/7 W	Lipid	5		
2/9 F			Demonstrations	
2/12 M	Lipid	5		
2/14 W	Protein	6		
2/16 F			Vegetarianism	234–242
2/19 M	Protein	6		
2/21 W	**EXAMINATION 2**	**4–6**		
2/23 F			Vitamin Supplements	344–349
2/26 M	Fluid and Electrolytes	7		
2/28 W	Fluid and Electrolytes	7		
3/2 F			Dietary Project	
3/5 M	Antioxidants	8		
3/7 W	Antioxidants	8		
3/9 F			Eating Disorders	Ch. 13
3/12-16	**SPRING BREAK**			
3/19 M	Bone Health	9		
3/21 W	Bone Health	9		
3/23 F			Obesity	Ch. 11
3/26 M	**EXAMINATION 3**	**7–9**		
3/28 W	Energy/Blood Health	10		
3/30 F			Ergogenic Aids	512–516

Date	Lecture Topic	Text Chapter	Discussion Topic	Text Pages
4/2 M	Energy/Blood Health	10		
4/4 W	Weight Control	11		
4/6 F	**SPRING RECESS**			
4/9 M	Physical Activity	12		
4/11 W	Physical Activity	12		
4/13 F			Food Safety	Ch. 14
4/16 M	**EXAMINATION 4**	**10–12**		
4/18 W	Food Safety	14		
4/20 F			Breastfeeding	Ch. 15
4/23 M	Pregnancy/Infancy	15		
4/25 W	Adolescence/Old Age	16		
4/27 F			Infant Growth	Ch. 15
5/2 Wed	**FINAL EXAMINATION**		**2:45-4:45 pm**	

Teaching Micronutrients: An Alternative Approach
continued from page 127

engaged in this material and it seemed more relevant as well. Let's face it, we don't often see deficiency diseases for thiamin, riboflavin, etc., so it may be better to spend that limited time teaching more relevant material. Now as I teach Principles of Nutrition, I use a very similar model.

The Model

I start out by introducing vitamins and minerals and discussing similarities and differences. I also introduce the concepts of toxicity and deficiency as well as bioavailability. In this introduction, I highlight one vitamin and mineral as an example of a nutrient in each classification. Usually I discuss vitamin A as my vitamin example and iodine as my mineral example because deficiencies of these nutrients worldwide are well documented, allowing me to bring in an international perspective. I take this opportunity to show students videos from UNICEF highlighting fortification and educational campaigns to overcome these deficiencies in parts of Africa as well as China and Ecuador. After this segment, I discuss vitamins and minerals as they relate to energy production, antioxidant activity, bone health, blood health, and blood pressure regulation. In the antioxidant segment, I introduce cancer and discuss its initiation and promotion. This topic also allows me to introduce the concept of phytochemicals and their possible role in disease prevention. When discussing blood pressure regulation, I give the students a chance to adjust a diet to meet the DASH (Dietary Approaches to Stop Hypertension) guidelines. The bone health unit includes a case study of an individual with multiple risk factors for osteoporosis. There are certainly other examples of vitamins and minerals impacting bodily functions that could be taught as well. For example, I have often thought of adding a segment on micronutrients and eye health.

Benefits

Using this system, I find that I include most of the information outlined in the traditionally organized textbook, but in a different format. Students seem to respond better to this organization by bodily function and it highlights the fact that vitamins and minerals work synergistically. I also clearly point out that we are just choosing a few examples of bodily functions that require vitamins and minerals so that students realize that we have truly just touched the surface. While I don't see as many sets of flashcards as I look out over the room, I do get more questions and discussion from my students. Equally important is the fact that I have a lot more fun teaching the material now that I have adopted this alternative format. ■

SERVICE LEARNING IN A HUMAN NUTRITION COURSE

Bonnie Wood, University of Maine at Presque Isle
wood@polaris.umpi.maine.edu

A goal of my one-semester Human Nutrition (Biology 300) course is to actively engage students in the learning of human nutrition. I emphasize that students *use* facts about nutrition instead of simply memorizing them. The students in this course represent a variety of majors including Elementary and Secondary Education, Physical Education Teaching, Athletic Training, Fitness/Wellness, Health Education, and Biology. I designed a service learning project to foster a lifelong interest in nutrition among both students and their volunteer partners; to prepare the students to make effective dietary choices for themselves, and to teach others to do the same; and to help students acquire thinking skills they can use in other life endeavors.

Preparation

Before the semester begins, I obtain approval for this project from the Institutional Review Board for the Protection of Human Subjects (IRB) at the University of Maine at Presque Isle. Next, I solicit volunteers with an e-mail to all University of Maine at Presque Isle employees in which I offer a "free nutritional assessment" and briefly explain the service learning project. More than enough people volunteer and I usually generate a waiting list for next year's course.

The Project

During the first weeks of the semester, students learn about the components of a healthful diet, the major nutrients, and how to interpret food labels. They evaluate their own diet and energy balance while acquiring this knowledge. To complete a stepwise nutritional assessment of themselves, students use and become comfortable with one of several computerized dietary analysis and scoring programs.

At mid-semester, I pair each student with a volunteer service learning partner and spend one class teaching them about IRB policies and guidelines as well as procedures to follow during the project. I emphasize the necessity of meticulous

Great Ideas! IN TEACHING NUTRITION

A BENJAMIN CUMMINGS PUBLICATION FOR NUTRITION INSTRUCTORS
VOLUME 1

TABLE OF CONTENTS

Innovative Teaching Strategies
Teaching Micronutrients: An Alternative Approach 127
Amy Allen-Chabot
Anne Arundel Community College
Service Learning in a Human Nutrition Course 128
Bonnie Wood
University of Maine at Presque Isle
Active Learning
Collaborative Group Projects 129
Sally Weerts
University of North Florida
How Bad is Fast Food, Really? 129
Frank Hendrick
Eastern Connecticut State University
Critical Thinking
Evaluating Popular Diets 130
Amy Allen-Chabot
Anne Arundel Community College
Personalizing the Diet and Health Connection 131
Janet B. Anderson
Utah State University
In-Class Activities
Consumer Investigation Project 132
Karen L. Smith, Washington College
Activities and Demonstrations for BasicConsumer Nutrition 132
Mary Ellen Clark
Monroe Community College
Interactive Nutrition Activities 133
Kate Brennan Shuey
Monroe Community College
Technology
Online Tour of a USDA Energy Metabolism Research Facility 133
Amy Allen-Chabot
Anne Arundel Community College
Food, Fitness, and Fun 134
Nancy Tress
University of Pittsburgh at Titusville

ABOUT THIS NEWSLETTER

Great Ideas in Teaching is published as a service to nutrition instructors. We welcome contributed articles and suggestions for future issues. Please contact us at nutrition@aw.com.

Welcome to the premier issue of Great Ideas in Teaching Nutrition. Even as a newcomer to nutrition, Benjamin Cummings has been fortunate to work with a talented and enthusiastic group of authors, reviewers, class-testers, and educators as we have produced learning materials for your students. In working with them, we are always impressed with the wide variety of "great ideas" that they bring into the classroom each term. This brief compilation of teaching ideas for nutrition is a sampling of your colleagues' pedagogical insights. We hope you will receive this newsletter as a measure of our commitment to supporting fine teaching—first through our textbooks and ancillary materials, but also by means of our technology and product in-services, and most recently, selected Benjamin Cummings Nutrition Forums for nutrition instructors.

Please join us in thanking the educators who took the time to contribute their ideas to this newsletter. May their great ideas be a source of inspiration to you and your students!

Innovative Teaching Strategies

TEACHING MICRONUTRIENTS: AN ALTERNATIVE APPROACH

Amy Allen-Chabot, Anne Arundel Community College
amallenchabot@aacc.edu

Back in the pre-Jurassic period, I took my first Nutrition class. Shortly after we began the section on vitamins and minerals, I realized that flash cards were the way to go! I made a card for each nutrient and listed sources and functions on the back. While I readily memorized all this information, I didn't retain much of it. Furthermore, I had no idea how much more information I hadn't even been exposed to. I finished the class thinking every micronutrient had only two or three functions in the body and a mere handful of food sources.

During my Ph.D. program at the University of Maryland (UMD), I was first exposed to a different way of teaching this material. Rather than presenting each micronutrient separately, faculty teaching the Principles of Nutrition courses at UMD grouped the vitamins and minerals based on common functions. Specifically, they discussed vitamins and minerals as they relate to blood health, bone health, antioxidant function, energy metabolism, etc. Though I was a bit resistant to this new organization of the material, I quickly became a believer. Students appeared to be more

continued on page 128

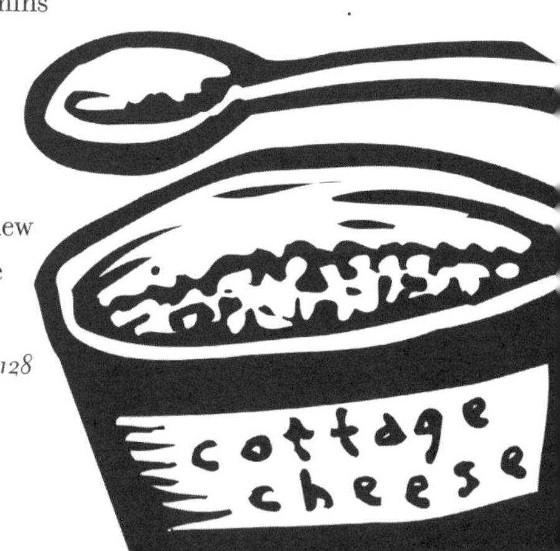

How Bad is Fast Food, Really?
continued from page 129

something than by simply hearing or reading about it. Active learning facilitates student retention of the desired information and improves their ability to apply it. I use a "discovery" method for two of the projects in my Foundations of Health Related Fitness class that serve to get students actively engaged with the topic of nutrition. Recent media coverage of the growth of obesity in society, increases in diabetes, and the recent lawsuits against McDonalds provided a good backdrop for the investigations I asked students to undertake.

The first project was a nutritional scavenger hunt, of sorts, at fast food restaurants in the local area. Students worked in pairs and had to plan two days of eating only fast food for breakfast, lunch, and dinner. The goal for the first day's diet plan was to find the *best* of the possible choices from the listed fast food menu. The second day's meal plan was to find the *worst* choices possible. In addition, bonus points were to be awarded to the group that "won" either of the two meal plans, so students had an incentive to dig through the menus and be creative.

Each student team had to identify the total calories, calories from fat, sodium, carbohydrates, and protein for each individual meal as well as for the entire day. Other stipulations were:

- The meal plan had to be realistic in what was being consumed.
- No restaurant could be used for more than one meal.
- Meal plans could be "super-sized."

The other students in the class were given the opportunity to vote down any meal plan that they felt was unrealistic. This meant that a meal might not be considered "realistic" if it consisted of four burgers, three shakes, and three large fries just to increase the calories and "win" the bonus points.

After the "scavenger hunt," student groups presented the data for their best and worst meal plans to the class. Because numerous restaurants could be selected, the meal plans were widely different. Many students were shocked when they heard the nutritional descriptions of meals that most of them had ordered at some time in the past. They also realized that many of the restaurants routinely advertise these same meals as a good option for people with a busy schedule. A side effect of the activity was that students started to understand the concept of portion size. In looking at the nutrition labels, they began to realize that an "order" at one of these restaurants would be considered more than one serving (e.g., a 20 oz. soda = 2.5 servings).

In order to incorporate the fitness and lifestyle component into the assignment, a second project, done in class, built on the data students had collected. This next step was to determine the exercise necessary to balance the diet identified in each of their meal plans.

This activity is a fun and competitive way for students to discover the real facts about fast food and the long-term impact of a diet built around fast food establishments. It is not designed to cast blame on the fast food industry but to help students make as healthy a choice as possible when they eat occasionally at these restaurants. It prompts the learner to "discover the truth" about diet and exercise and may help them make better choices. ■

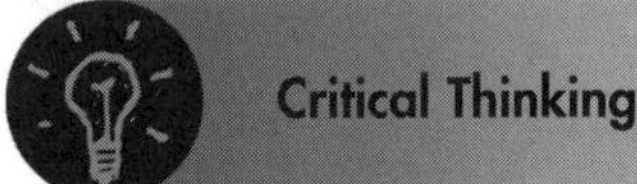

Critical Thinking

EVALUATING POPULAR DIETS

Amy Allen-Chabot, Anne Arundel Community College amallenchabot@aacc.edu

Teaching critical thinking skills is one of the toughest and most important challenges we face as educators. I find it is especially difficult in introductory science classes because students lack the basic knowledge necessary to think critically about complex issues. One of the critical thinking activities that I have had success with is the assessment of popular diets. This is an activity I do in the last third of the semester so that students can draw on the knowledge they have gained up to that point.

To introduce this activity, I ask students to spend a few days thinking about how they might evaluate a popular diet, based on all that they have learned about nutrients and weight management. Once the students have had a chance to think about this, I have an in-class brainstorming session where we list appropriate criteria for evaluation of weight loss diets. Students usually identify some of the following criteria:

- Is it missing any essential nutrients?
- Does it provide too much of any nutrients?

confidentiality regarding information about volunteer participants.

The service learning project is completed outside of class. Additional topics on human nutrition fill the remaining weeks of the semester's class meetings.

In lieu of a final exam, students submit a final paper that is a detailed nutritional assessment of their service learning partner. A copy of this assessment is given to the service learning partner to keep. To thank the partners and to celebrate the end of the course, the students plan and prepare a healthful meal for the volunteers. Displayed on the buffet table are "Nutrition Facts" labels that students prepared for each recipe or food item, so this event is both enjoyable and educational. ■

Active Learning

COLLABORATIVE GROUP PROJECTS

Sally E. Weerts, University of North Florida
sweerts@unf.edu

For many years, group projects have been a part of introductory nutrition courses. Designed to allow collaboration among students in lecture courses of 50 or more, group projects can also work in courses with fewer students.

When asked about the benefits of group projects, most students respond that meeting others in a large lecture is most beneficial to them. From the instructor's point of view, encouraging individuals to become more actively involved with the content is most valuable. Although the instructor loses teaching time, the students gain peer-learning time. And because group projects in my course are always conducted during the class period before the exam, learning from multiple sources may enhance academic performance.

I assign four projects for the semester, with each project worth up to fifteen points.

Forming the Groups

Students form groups of 3–4 each, and select one person to be the "leader of the day." Each person should be the leader at least once. The leader chooses the topic (by placing the number of his/her group by the topic), completes the evaluation form, and hands in the evaluation form as his/her group goes to the front of the room to present their project.

The best way to summarize the experience of group projects is to share the course handout.

Group Projects

The objective of each of your four group projects is to examine and represent a topic more deeply or broadly than it is covered in lecture. *Examine* means to discover what more can be known about the topic. *Represent* means to present more about the topic so that you and your classmates can know more than the lecture taught you. *More deeply* means adding more content about the same things that lecture covered. *More broadly* means adding new content about the topic that lecture did not include.

For example, think among yourselves about the topic you have selected. What is missing from your understanding about the topic? Brainstorm ideas. Learn from each other. Use your text as a reference. Ask the professor for clarification.

Topics

Project 1 DRIs, Food Guide Pyramid, food labels, exchange system, sugars, starch, or fiber

Project 2 Amino acids, fatty acids and glycerol, fats in food, protein in food, fat functions, or protein functions

Project 3 The digestion, absorption, and transport of carbohydrates; the digestion, absorption, and transport of protein; the digestion, absorption, and transport of fat; loss of weight from body fat; low-calorie diets; or metabolism

Project 4 Functions and food sources of water soluble vitamins, functions and food sources of fat soluble vitamins, major minerals, or trace minerals

Presentations

Present your organized thoughts about the topic to the class. Topics may be presented in a variety of ways:

Artistic – a poster	Written summary
Dramatic – a play	Role play
Comedy sketch	Game show

Everyone in your group will participate in some equal way during your group's presentation. Your group has 2–3 minutes to present your group project (and the hook will help you off the stage at 3 minutes).

Evaluations

Self evaluate your group's representation. Score yourselves and answer the question on the back of the evaluation that your instructor will bring to each group while you are preparing for your presentation. ■

HOW BAD IS FAST FOOD, REALLY?

Frank Hendrick, Eastern Connecticut State University hendrickf@easternct.edu

Incorporating experiential education into the classroom or learning environment is very important. Many students learn more easily by doing

continued on page 130

PERSONALIZING THE DIET AND HEALTH CONNECTION

continued from page 131

Students report this assignment as being the motivator to make lifestyle changes. Many students are surprised to learn about their familial diseases—many had no idea that their father had hypertension or what their grandmother or grandfather had died from. Many students have reported that this assignment was a wake-up call and prompted them to action. We have found that this simple exercise gives students a personal reason to make lifestyle changes—it gives them the "why" for behavior modification. ■

In-Class Activities

CONSUMER INVESTIGATION PROJECT

Karen L. Smith, Washington College
ksmith2@washcoll.edu

Here's a project students have found very informative—both as researchers/presenters and as listeners to the oral reports.

Each student selects three versions of the same product (for example, yogurt, chips, cereals, energy bars, crackers, breads, soups, cookies, etc.) and does a thorough investigation of the products using the label information. They then write up a comparison of the ingredients (calories, protein, fat, carbohydrates, price, etc.) and give an oral presentation to the class, explaining what's good and/or bad about each product (high fat content, chemical additives, too much sodium, etc.). They also provide a written handout with the label information and all ingredients on it so classmates can follow the figures. Their report also involves some math as they compare the three products with their percentages of fat, carbohydrates, and protein. Students can either compare the product with two other flavors, or two other brands of the same flavor. The handout below contains the label information for a yogurt comparison.

Light & Lively Black Cherry Yogurt
240 cal/8oz/$.67

Protein	9 gm	36 cal	15%
Carbohydrate	44 gm	176 cal	73%
Fat	3 gm	27 cal	11%

Ingredients: low fat milk, sugar, skim milk, etc.

Their discussion includes best value for price and ingredients, whether a "serving" is actually what most people would eat (only 2 Oreos = a serving? Get real!), and how many calories they are really likely to eat.

I don't require them to purchase or taste the products, but many of the students do, and some share them with their dorm mates for a taste test. Some even pass brown paper bags (unlabeled) around the class for a taste test and have us choose which we like best before they give us the "scoop" on the ingredients. For some, this is the first time they have ever looked at a label! ■

ACTIVITIES AND DEMONSTRATIONS FOR BASIC CONSUMER NUTRITION

Mary Ellen Clark, Monroe Community College
mclark@monroecc.edu

In-Class Portion Estimation Activity

I set up different types of foods, such as peanuts, cereal, milk, raisins, snack foods, etc., on separate tables. Some of the foods are real and some are models of food. I have students estimate portion sizes, using cups, teaspoons, tablespoons, and so on for reference. I also ask them to estimate the calories in each of the portions.

After the students have finished their activity, I provide them with the actual portion sizes and calories for each food. I also have them answer some questions related to the activity. I ask them if they tend to over- or underestimate their portions, and what they used for a reference to help them determine the portion size. I ask this in particular because many people tend to use restaurant portions as standard portions.

Sugar in Soft Drinks Demonstration

I start this demonstration with a clear glass of water. I ask students how many teaspoons of sugar are found in a can of soda. When I add 10 teaspoons and show them all of that sugar in the bottom of the glass, they are blown away. One could do the same demonstration for juice drinks or other drinks for comparison.

Fat in Fast Foods Demonstration

I pass vials of fat that are found in different fast foods. NASCO or another company produces these

- Is it so different from an average individual's normal eating pattern that compliance is unlikely?
- Will the person learn new and healthful ways of eating so that they can *keep* the weight off?
- Is it expensive?
- Does it provide a kcalorie deficit? (Does it result in a person eating fewer kcalories than they are using?)
- Is it too low in kcalories?
- Does it include unnecessary restrictions?
- Are the credentials of the person promoting the diet sound?
- Is the approach supported by our current body of scientific evidence?
- Does the diet make reasonable claims regarding weight loss?

I then list a number of popular diets on the board and ask students to sign up for the diet they would like to study. Using that "preference" list, I form groups ranging from 2 to 4 students and ask them to use the criteria identified in class to evaluate the chosen diet. Students are instructed to use several sources and to cite all sources used. A sheet describing how to reference Web sites is provided.

Students have two weeks to complete this assessment. During the second week, I give students 20 minutes in class to share their information with group members and discuss the information in relation to the class- generated criteria. They can then write up one assignment per group, distributing the work accordingly. In addition, I ask students to complete a group member evaluation form that asks them to evaluate the effort of each group member, including themselves, based on the percent of total work. For example, a student in a 4-member group would list each member, including themselves, and give each member 25%. I stress that this percentage is an indication of effort, not ability, since someone that has been on a given diet will certainly know more about the diet than fellow classmates. I have found that individuals are very honest about their level of participation.

Students seem to enjoy this activity, despite the fact that they generally express a dislike for group activities that require outside group member coordination. After all assignments are turned in, we discuss some of the more popular diets and students appreciate being able to contribute and share their newly-acquired expertise. ■

PERSONALIZING THE DIET AND HEALTH CONNECTION

Janet B. Anderson, Utah State University
janet.anderson@usu.edu

Motivating college freshmen to change their lifestyle (diet and activity) to improve their health is as challenge, but extremely important. It is easy to give the statistics:

- Of the ten leading causes of death in the US, four causes are directly related to nutrition. These four conditions account for about two-thirds of the nation's two million deaths each year.
- Two out of every three adults in the US are overweight or obese, which is emerging as the most important contributor to ill health.

It is not, however, easy to motivate students to make lifestyle changes to prevent these chronic diseases.

My nutrition course, a general education life science course, is designed to teach the scientific principles of nutrition and their application. Teaching the application is the challenge because we have over 400 students in each section. We don't have recitations, all assignments are completed online, and students perceive themselves as invincible. We developed a series of comprehensive diet analysis assignments to teach them how their personal dietary intake compared to recommendations, but we weren't able to motivate most of them to make changes in their lifestyle now, not later in life.

Motivating Students

Our solution was to teach diet and health as a capstone unit and incorporate an online diet and health assignment. This assignment requires students to list the following information about their parents and grandparents: diseases they had, the age at which they died and cause of death, and whether or not they are/were obese or overweight. Students list their personal BMI, interpretation of their BMI (e.g., normal weight, underweight, overweight, or obese), and any chronic diseases they have. The students are asked to evaluate each of their familial diseases and determine if there is a nutrition link to each disease. Students are then asked to list the lifestyle changes that they need to make to reduce their personal risk of suffering from their familial diseases.

continued on page 132

vials. They are effective at showing the students the amounts of fat found in fast foods or junk food.

Current News Discussions

I collect articles from popular health magazines, newspapers, and nutrition newsletters and have students read an article in a small group. They are then asked to answer some questions and share the information from their article with the class. This can be done with articles related to a single topic or to a specific textbook chapter. This activity can be tough if students are shy, but if the articles are interesting, the discussion gets started and is interesting for everyone. ■

INTERACTIVE NUTRITION ACTIVITIES

Kate Brennan Shuey
Monroe Community College

Here are two in-class activities I have tried.

Portioning Activity

Since I implemented this activity, student grades on diet analysis projects have increased.

Stations spaced throughout the room are equipped with food samples and measuring tools such as cups, spoons, and food scales. Students, in groups of three, rotate among the stations and complete the pertinent questions about each station. Remaining students work on a different activity in the back of the room. Following is a sampling of the station contents and tasks.

- Dry/cooked rice and dry/canned fruit: Measure one-half cup of each and compare the number of calories in them.
- Granola/raisin and crispy rice-type cereal: Measure and weigh one cup of each and compare them.

Soy Milk Sampling

I provide chilled samples of vanilla and chocolate soymilk to students when they are discussing alternatives to animal-based proteins, functional foods, and food sanitation. Five to ten percent of students try the products and more than 80 percent of those students make favorable comments such as "This isn't bad," "I like it," or "This is good for my chocolate fix."

Body Model Manipulation

Two body model torsos containing the digestive system organs are placed on carts in opposite corners of the room. Each model comes with index cards containing the names of digestive organs. There is also a photograph of actual human digestive organs on each cart. Students approach the models in groups of four or five. Their task is to put the index cards in order from mouth to anus while removing the organs from the body model. They discuss the function of each organ, using their text as a reference, view the photographs, then replace the organs. ■

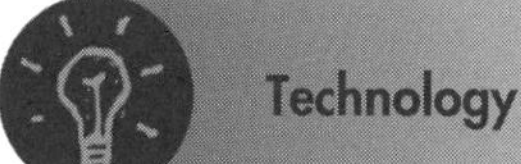

Technology

ONLINE TOUR OF A USDA ENERGY METABOLISM RESEARCH FACILITY

Amy Allen-Chabot, Anne Arundel Community College
amallenchabot@aacc.edu

When teaching about kcalories in food and kcalories needed by individuals, would you like to be able to show students how kcaloric expenditure is measured? When talking about clinical trials and feeding studies, would you like to be able to show students a real research-level feeding kitchen? When talking about bone mass or body fat percentage, would you like to be able to show students how this might be measured in a research study? Thanks to the Internet, your students can now see all of this without leaving their desks.

With the help of a small college funded grant, we were able to produce a streaming audio/streaming video online field trip of the USDA Human Research Center in Beltsville, Maryland. You can access our online virtual field trip of the USDA research center by going to *http://www2.aacc.edu/nutrition* and clicking on "Virtual field trip of the Beltsville Human Nutrition Research Center." (Please note: In order to access the field trip, a student must have "Realplayer" on their computer. This can be downloaded for free from the link on the field trip Web page.)

The field trip allows students to see the indirect calorimetry room, the DEXA (dual energy X-ray absorptiometry) machine, and the feeding kitchen. The DEXA machine uses low dose X-rays to differentiate between fat mass, lean body mass, and bone. Throughout the tour, Dr. Seale, a USDA human nutrition researcher, describes the facility and some of the research conducted at this extraordinary human research lab. A set of questions at the end of the online field trip can be printed or copied by students, answered using information gleaned from the field trip, and handed in as homework or as an extra credit assignment. ■

FOOD, FITNESS, AND FUN

Nancy Tress, University of Pittsburgh at Titusville
ntress@pitt.edu

At the University of Pittsburgh at Titusville, we have added a nutrition course to fulfill a science requirement for our business students. To be eligible for graduation, these students must complete a science course that includes a lab component. There are several lab courses offered on our campus, but none are designed for nonmajors. To meet this graduation requirement, we felt the need to offer a new course appropriate for a mixed student population and with a lab that would be cost-effective. A nutrition course seemed a logical choice because the subject matter is relevant both for science majors and nonmajors.

The Nutrition Lab

One aspect of the nutrition lab is an assessment of the eating habits of each of the students. A software program called Fitday is used to perform this analysis. This program is available for use at *http: www.fitday.com*. Students can either use the program online free of charge or purchase a copy for a nominal fee. On the first day of lab, students are asked to keep a journal of the food they eat for the next seven days. They then enter that data into Fitday and are able to print out a nutritional assessment that includes the amount of fat, protein, and carbohydrates consumed. They are also able to assess any deficiencies in vitamin and mineral intake. The students then use this information to determine what alterations to their diet are needed. Once these changes are implemented, the students continue to use the Fitday program to track their progress. Every four weeks students hand in an assessment to show progress made in their eating habits.

The Taste Test

Another aspect of the nutrition lab is designed to help students modify their busy lifestyles to include better nutritional choices. One of the most popular activities in the lab, the taste test, is designed to help students think about different food options and encourage them to try different recipes. We have a taste test at the end of lab every four weeks.

For the taste test, each student chooses one of the four dates to bring a dish of their choice. They can bring anything they want as long as it is a "healthy" choice. This will work for both dormitory students and commuter students. The selections have included non-cooking options, such as baked potato chips or pretzels, drink options such as fruit smoothies, and home-cooked entrees ranging from broccoli casserole to vegetarian chili. Generally, there are six to eight students providing different foods for each taste test.

The first semester this course was taught, there was no theme associated with each taste test and a wide variety of foods was offered each time. This semester the taste tests were done on four theme nights: Superbowl, On The Go, The Breakfast Club, and Mardi Gras.

Feedback

Both methods have been hugely successful. The taste test was so popular last year that the students asked to have a picnic at the end of the semester where everyone brought some healthy contribution. This is a great way for students to get new ideas or modify their own recipes to make them healthier. As each student presented their taste test contribution, I asked that they email me a copy of the recipe they used or developed. I then put all the recipes together into a cookbook that the students received at the end of the semester.

In conclusion, it is possible to construct a lab for a nutrition class that is affordable, relevant, and enjoyable. The lab adds a practical experience that supplements the lecture material by teaching students how to assess their nutrition and to adjust their behavior accordingly. The lab component has helped to make this course an extremely popular choice among science majors as well as nonmajors. ■

Eating Healthy on a Budget
continued from page 135

chips, and other big bag snack items are fabulous bargains compared to the costs of fruit, vegetables, and other healthy foods. These are considered to be expensive choices. I smile inside and say, "Ok… let's have a Shopping Face-Off to see how truly expensive it is to eat healthy." Then the fun begins.

The Shopping Face-Off

I ask for four volunteers to compete on a two-person shopping team in the front of the classroom to see how much food can be purchased with a budget of $10. One of the team members is the "Shopper." The other is the "Checkout Person" and is given a calculator. Each team is provided with a large brown grocery bag containing food items. One bag is labeled *Healthy Foods* and the other is labeled *Could Be Better*. The competition begins.

The first Shopper pulls out a one-pound box of Prince pasta ($.99) from the *Healthy Foods* bag, and the Checkout Person enters this amount into the team's calculator. The other team's Shopper reaches in their *Could Be Better* bag and grabs a petite bag of Pepperidge Farm Milano Cookies ($2.99). This amount is entered into their calculator. "Wow!" I say. "Who knew that a cute little pouch of about a dozen cookies would cost more than a pound of pasta." They laugh. The contest continues with similar comments between each round of purchases. However, as you can see from the contents of the bags listed below, there are only three rounds of shopping before the *Could Be Better* team could have been, well, better, when it came to getting the most out of their $10 budget.

Team Results

Healthy Foods Shopping Bag		*Could Be Better* Shopping Bag	
Prince Pasta, 1 lb	$.99	Pepperidge Farm Milano Cookies, 15 cookies	$2.99
Bumble Bee Tuna, Chunk Lite, canned	$.69	M & M Candy, large bag, 21 oz	$4.29
Columbo Lite Yogurt	$.67	Haagen Dazs Ice Cream, 1 pint	$2.99
Birds Eye Green Beans, frozen, 1 lb	$1.00		
Libby's Lite Peaches, canned,15 oz	$.99		
Quaker Oatmeal, 42 oz	$3.99		
Progresso Black Beans, canned, 19 oz	$.50		
Bananas, small bunch	$1.25		
Totals	**$10.08**		**$10.27**

After the third round of the Face-Off, the *Healthy Foods* team continues pulling items from their bag, dramatically illustrating the point that $10 can go farther in the grocery store. I then point out that there are not only more than twice as many items in the *Healthy Foods* bag than the other, but that these healthier foods also provide selections from each of the basic five food groups. A mere $10 can be stretched to cover a bounty of healthy foods.

I have found that this classroom exercise is an entertaining way to teach students that eating healthy doesn't have to break the bank. In fact, it also illustrates that a diet rich in sweets and treats can quickly drain their wallets. ■

PRACTICAL ACTIVITIES FOR TEACHING THE EXCHANGE SYSTEM

Teresa Johnson, Troy University School of Nursing
tjohnson@troy.edu

A fundamental basic nutrition skill is estimating the calorie content and grams of fat, carbohydrate, and protein in a meal or food. The Exchange System for Meal Planning is the vehicle for that instruction. However, many students fail to see the practical value of the system, as most texts do not provide learning activities that use Exchange System information. I developed three learning activities that use the Exchange System presented in the appendix of the textbook. To minimize the amount of time needed to grade these instruments, I use self-graded online exams that are developed and posted in Blackboard. These are automatically graded and posted in the electronic grade book, and students have instant feedback on their work. The exam is identical to the activities. This gives students ample time to complete the sheets, then go to the computer to enter their answers. These activities can be utilized in both online and Web-enhanced courses. The three part activity follows.

Editor's Note: The following tables are excerpted versions of the activity.The complete versions can be viewed on the Web at www.aw-bc.com/greatideas.

The Exchange System for Menu Planning Activity

The Exchange System for Menu Planning is a useful tool for estimating total calories and grams of carbohydrate, fat, and protein in a single food or meal. Print this sheet and using the information presented in Table 2.8,

Great Ideas! IN TEACHING NUTRITION

A BENJAMIN CUMMINGS PUBLICATION FOR NUTRITION INSTRUCTORS
VOLUME 2

TABLE OF CONTENTS

Active Learning
Eating Healthy on a Budget 135
Joan Salge Blake
Boston University
Practical Activities for Teaching the Exchange System 136
Teresa Johnson
Troy University School of Nursing
Two Teaching Strategies for an Interactive Nutrition Class 137
Rosa Polanco-Paula
Miami-Dade Community College
Using Real Models to Introduce Life Cycle Topics in Nutrition 138
Tish Erdmann
Middle Tennessee State University

Critical Thinking
Heart Risk Screening Activity 138
Ruth Reilly and Jesse Stabile Morrell
University of New Hampshire
Tasting: A Missing Element in Nutrition? 139
Ken Bourgoin
Valencia Community College
A Treat Project 140
Carol Ribner
New Hampshire Community Technical College

Web-Enhanced Activities
Using Web-Enhanced Tools to Teach Cultural Nutrition Practices 141
Teresa Johnson
Troy University School of Nursing
Engaging Students on the Web and in the Classroom 141
Allison Miner
Prince George's Community College

COMPANION WEB SITE

Resources related to this issue can be found on the Web at www.aw-bc.com/greatideas.

ABOUT THIS NEWSLETTER

Great Ideas in Teaching is published as a service to nutrition instructors. We welcome contributed articles and suggestions for future issues. Please contact us at nutrition@aw.com.

Welcome to the second issue of **Great Ideas!***, brought to you by the nutrition publishing team at Benjamin Cummings. Once again, your colleagues have taken the time to share some of the innovative ways in which they enliven the nutrition classroom and motivate students to connect what they learn to their eating habits and personal health. In this issue, you will find in-class activities, extra-credit projects, and ideas for using Web-based tools such as Blackboard to engage your students in different ways.*

New to this issue are references to online materials that support the articles you see in print. In cases where space did not allow for the complete text of a handout, sample, or rubric, you can jump to the Companion Web Site (www.aw-bc.com/greatideas) to find it. No passwords are required for access to the Companion Web Site—just type the url into your browser and look for the link to the **Great Ideas!** *newsletter for Nutrition.*

We at Benjamin Cummings appreciate the talent and enthusiasm of the authors, reviewers, class-testers, and educators that we work with and are pleased to be able to share some of their "great ideas" with you. Please join us in thanking the contributors to this issue for making this possible. May their ideas be a source of "nutrition" for your own teaching!

Active Learning

EATING HEALTHY ON A BUDGET

Joan Salge Blake, Boston University
salge@bu.edu

It's 8 am and the students are filing into my non-majors, Introduction to Nutrition classroom. An athletic-looking man walks in with a 20-ounce container, which is taller than his notebook, of Starbucks Caramel Macchiato ($3.68) in one hand and a Power Bar ($2.25) in the other. The woman behind him is slurping a Dunkin Donuts Iced Latte ($3.69) and nibbling at a Crumb Cake Muffin ($1.49) that is so large that it dwarfs her entire hand. Here you have the college student's answer to breakfast. (We, as nutrition professors, were put on Earth to save these individuals.)

Since this morning's lecture is about the cost of eating healthy, I couldn't have planted more perfect examples of how college students overpay for trendy, designer foods. I start the lecture by polling the class, "How many of you think that it's expensive to eat a healthy diet?" More than 75 percent of the hands go up. Mentally, I am smiling—they took the bait. "Why do you think that?" I ask in a fake puzzled tone. The typical response is that fast food "Value Meals,"

continued on page 136

Table 2.9, and Appendix F, complete the following exercises. When you have completed each section, select the Exam button and complete the Exchange System Exam using the activity sheet as a reference.

Activity 1. Assign the food to its proper Exchange System List in the table below. (Some items might be a combination food or a 'free' food.)

Table 2.8

Food Item	Starch	Vegetable	Fruit	Meat	Milk	Fat	Free	Other Carbohydrate
Pretzels								
Cantaloupe								
Plain yogurt								
Individual pan pizza								
Orange juice								
Baked beans								
Corn								
Green beans								
...								
Fat Free Milk								
Collard Greens								

Activity 2. Using Exchange System Values, determine the number of calories, grams of carbohydrate, grams of fat, and grams of protein in the following meal and enter it in the table below. (Watch the serving sizes and number of servings.)

3 oz baked chicken (medium fat meat)
1/3 cup cooked pasta
1/2 cup cooked broccoli
1 oz swiss cheese
1 roll
2 teaspoons margarine
1/2 cup mandarin oranges
1/2 cup skim milk

Table 2.9

Menu Item	Calories	Carb Grams	Fat Grams	Protein Grams
Chicken				
Pasta				
Broccoli				
Swiss cheese				
Roll				
Margarine				
Oranges				
Skim milk				
Totals				

Activity 3. Mr. Smith is a diabetic who is learning the Carbohydrate Counting System to manage his blood glucose levels. In this system, a person injects a set amount of short-acting insulin to respond to blood glucose levels that will rise after consuming carbohydrates. His doctor has prescribed 0.5 units of insulin to be injected for every 15 grams of carbohydrate consumed. How many units of insulin should Mr. Smith inject after eating the meal presented in Activity 2?

Total grams carbohydrate: ______

Carbohydrate grams divided by 15 = ______ × 0.5 units insulin

Total units of insulin needed for this meal = ______ ■

TWO TEACHING STRATEGIES FOR AN INTERACTIVE NUTRITION CLASS

Rosa Polanco-Paula, Miami-Dade Community College
rpolanco@mdc.edu

Soliciting Student Participation

I conduct an interactive class that uses motivational interviewing language to solicit participation and provide feedback. I do this by asking questions throughout the class and using supporting statements such as "perhaps you would like to elaborate" or "I can certainly understand how you see it that way" instead of "You are wrong. Could someone help Jon Doe to explain the concept of complex carbohydrates?" This strategy stimulates participation and helps students not feel too embarrassed or timid to participate. To assess comprehension and train students to succeed in my exams, I ask questions in class as I would on the exams.

Extra Credit Projects

I also assign extra credit projects that are relevant to daily life. Here are five that I am using this semester:

1. Go to the site Mypyramid.gov and create your personalized pyramid, then contrast your current intake to the recommendation. Choose one thing you would like to change and evaluate the outcome.
2. Visit an ethnic restaurant and write a brief (1–3 page, typed) paper about your experience and the nutritional benefits of eating that particular cuisine.
3. View the documentary "Supersizeme" and critique it in terms of validity and nutrition message.
4. To learn more about proteins and vegetarian diets, follow a vegan diet for a day and write about the experience, and the challenges and rewards of following this diet.
5. Grocery Store Hunt: Find specific items (related to the current chapter) on food labels such as sugar alcohols, types of fat, additives, etc. ■

USING REAL MODELS TO INTRODUCE LIFE CYCLE TOPICS IN NUTRITION

Tish Erdmann, Middle Tennessee State University
lerdmann@mtsu.edu

This spring, I brought a variety of children into my Principles of Nutrition class to help introduce the chapters on Infancy, Toddlers, School-age Children, and Adolescents. I had over 70 students enrolled in the course, which is designed for non-majors. These students often have a high level of interest in the subject matter, but need learning formats other than lecture.

The Activity

The children who participated were boys and girls, ages 2, 6, 9, and 11. I divided the class up into four small sections and rotated the children (and in some cases their parents) among the groups. Each group had ten minutes to interview the child or parent about eating habits, physical activity, etc. Some of the younger children brought a letter they had written to describe their favorite foods. This helped overcome shyness on the part of both the children and the students. Having parents present assisted with communications for both the 2-and 6-year-olds.

Sample questions were given to the students, children, and parents to help stimulate initial conversations, but once the students warmed up, they began asking their own questions that made the interactions more natural and informative.

Findings and Benefits

After the activity, as we began the life cycle chapters, we were able to associate growth patterns with the real children we had seen in the classroom. Putting the image of a child in the minds of the students stimulated quality class discussion. Even the most reserved students could not resist the opportunity to get involved.

I was truly amazed at some of the student observations. They were able to make correlations between school physical education programs and levels of activity and fitness. They discovered the world of food jags and heard first-hand some of the frustrations parents experience. For more information about the activity, I invite you to contact me. ■

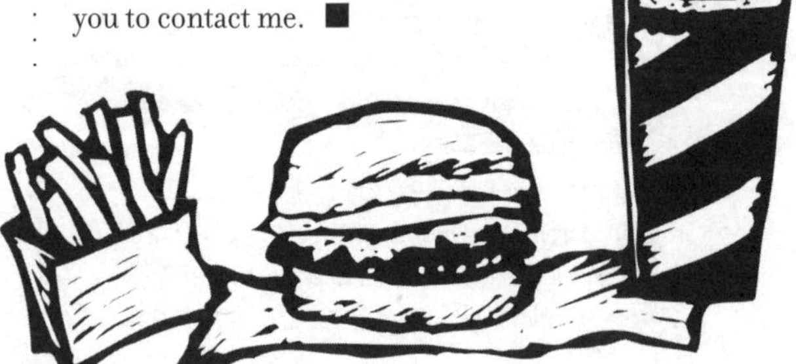

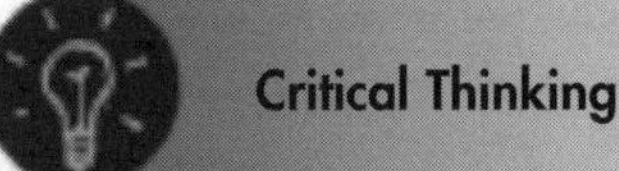

Critical Thinking

HEART RISK SCREENING ACTIVITY

Ruth A. Reilly and Jesse Stabile Morrell,
University of New Hampshire
ruth.reilly@unh.edu, jesse.morrell@unh.edu

Although students can relate to the topic of nutrition on a personal level, making every lecture interesting and relevant is still an ongoing challenge. In our introductory course we employ an innovative activity within the cardiovascular unit. It is designed to help students connect what they learn in lecture about evaluating personal cardiovascular risk to their own future health.

Even though heart disease is the leading cause of death in the United States, few college students perceive it as an important health risk. To engage students in the information as well as the relationship between current lifestyle choices and the development of chronic disease, we use a heart risk screening activity. The activity enhances student learning of the subject material as it motivates them to make healthier lifestyle choices.

The Screening

After the assignment is explained in class, students preschedule their screening appointment and are instructed to arrive at the testing site after a 12-hour fast. During the fifteen-minute appointment, trained technicians and graduate students measure blood pressure, waist circumference, blood lipids, and glucose. The efficiency and immediacy of the screening is facilitated by the Cholestech LDX® System, which measures the biochemical parameters from a finger stick within five minutes.

Formal Assessment Project

After the screening, students complete a formal assessment project outside of class. The project combines objective questions concerning the topic of heart disease with subjective questions related to the student's individual lifestyle and health parameters. In particular, students review their own risk factors for developing heart disease using screening results, personal and family medical history, height and weight, and dietary habits. Further, they are asked to identify lifestyle strategies that could decrease their risk. We also have them visit the Arizona Heart Institute's Web site (www.azheart.com) and conduct a risk factor analysis. This online resource incorporates educational resources personalized to the students' individual answers and provides the student with a score indicating their risk of developing heart disease. The National Heart, Lung, and Blood Institute's Web site is another online risk factor assessment option (www.nhlbi.nih.gov).

Student Feedback

By providing students with their own measurement values, we believe we have engaged them more effectively on the topic of heart disease. In addition to the fact that the vast majority (approximately 75 percent) have never had their blood lipids checked, students commented that the assignment truly raised their interest, and therefore comprehension, of the risk factors for heart disease. By moving beyond the information in lecture to make it relevant to their personal health, students are able to understand their own risk factors for heart disease. Ideally, this awareness will have a positive effect on their lifestyle practices. ■

TASTING: A MISSING ELEMENT IN NUTRITION?

Ken Bourgoin, Valencia Community College
kbourgoin@valenciacc.edu

Obviously "tasting" is not the total picture in a nutrition class. We Hospitality and Culinary students must have a significant amount of insight into the nutritional items they are buying and selling. But the key is "the emphasis!" The point is to emphasize the final linchpin of what the students may buy by *tasting*.

Putting food in your mouth involves the perceptions of aroma, taste, and texture. Your brain is registering these sensations in varying degrees of pleasure or displeasure. I have discovered that teaching the elements of taste and what food does in your mouth solidifies why specific flavor combinations hit or miss. First time Culinarian/Hospitality students learn not to alter the basics but find freedom in the reasons why such a recipe was created successfully in the first place. They then take that understanding of classical technique and test the limits of creativity with little or no mistakes in the final output. So how do you do a tasting within a class?

Most of the food and drink that I have tested in the classroom takes little effort in preparing or dividing. For example, chocolate peanut butter bars usually come in 4 or 6 packs. I divide the bars up, place them in numbered containers, and hide the packages the food came in. Generally students can guess what the product is when they see it, which establishes a preconceived idea in their brains. (Good or bad doesn't matter in Hospitality; if your consumers want the product you still have to educate yourself on the best to buy.)

Pass out plates, cups, or napkins and have the students number each food item according to the number on the container. (Please try not to let anyone taste if they have an allergy or intolerance for any of the items.) Before they taste, tell them you're going to ask two questions after each food item:

1. What sensations did it trigger in your mouth? (Notice the front, middle, and back of your mouth.)
2. What do you think is in it?

With liquids I ask them to swish the liquid in their mouth, like mouth wash, once from side to side, then swallow. This allows for a healthy gulp. Then I ask the questions:

1. What does the liquid taste like? (What does it remind you of?)
2. What did it do in your mouth from beginning to end?

The effects are amazing. The students can usually successfully tell you what some of the ingredients are. I then pull out the package and read the ingredients. With the chocolate peanut butter bars, I will mix healthy with less healthy version and get great responses. Sometimes it doesn't taste "in their minds" like it is supposed to taste to them in their mouth, which often relates to the textures found in some products. If some products require cooking I usually ask them, "Is there another way of cooking the product to promote one flavor over another and make a difference in the final outcome?" I encourage them not to tell me they hate it, although that happens, but what they could do to modify it to change the aspect they don't like.

The end result is they can start to make better educated assessments of the kinds of things they buy within the nutritional realm. Teach them not to just look at a product and assume it's OK. They need to follow through. I believe taste has been at the forefront of this revolution of new products. Healthy or less healthy, the products will stay on the shelves for one final reason only. Taste! ■

A TREAT PROJECT

Carol Ribner, New Hampshire Community Technical College
cribner@nhctc.edu

One of my classroom activities is to have students prepare a food item at home to bring to class for other class members to eat. The project is scheduled twice during the semester. The first treat project is due the week after we have completed chapters discussing carbs, lipids, and proteins; the second after vitamins and minerals. Students are given the instruction sheet below, a list of legally defined terms, and an example project. We cover the math in bits and pieces over the first few weeks. The math to arrive at percents and total calories and the commentary on the food is the focus — no computer programs are allowed.

After the feast (?), students are expected to discuss their food item, its calories, percent of various nutrients, and make a valid comment. I've had students prepare regular and low-fat versions of various food items and food items for those with special dietary needs (e.g., a banana yogurt drink which supplies electrolytes, simple carbs and is low in lactose for children with/recovering from gastroenteritis) as well as everyday items. We have some microwaves in the cafeteria for reheating, and I supply the plastic and paperware. The students seem to enjoy the break from the usual classroom lecture.

Treat Project

Guidelines

- Food items are to be prepared in advance by student(s) and brought to class for consumption, tasting, and evaluation by all members of the class.
- If the class is large (more than 24), students will work in pairs (division of labor is the responsibility of the students). There will be two exercises of this nature during the semester.
- Treats may be any item of food — soup, drink, appetizer, main course, veggie, dessert, or snack. *Only one of your food items can be a snack food/ junk food/dessert.* However, you do not have to make a treat that is considered a snack food, junk food, or dessert.

Written Report

The second part of the assignment consists of the recipe with instructions for preparation, as well as a breakdown of the calories and nutrients contributed by each ingredient per serving, i.e., what percentage of calories come from lipids, proteins, and carbohydrates. Include any kind of information that would be of interest to a consumer, i.e., amounts of sodium, simple sugar, fat (cholesterol, saturated fat, unsaturated fat), and complex carbohydrates. *Math calculations must be attached. Show all computations.* Source(s) of nutrition information must be cited.

Also include a commentary of the (un)worthiness of the food and how it does or should fit into the average diet. Comments may include remarks about the high or low quantity of particular nutrients with potential benefits or drawbacks, i.e., if the item contains lots of salt, perhaps it should be avoided by people with high blood pressure. If the item has lots of table (simple) sugar, it is a dentist's dream and diabetic's nightmare. Or, would you want your children to consume the food item on a regular basis?

Grading

This is a two-part assignment that will receive two separate grades. No partial grades will be awarded.You (or your partner) must do both parts of the assignment to get a grade. If you work with a partner who fails to do his/her part, both of you will receive the same low grade (0).

If you work with a partner, both names should appear on the written assignment. If you fail to complete the entire exercise correctly, your work will be returned to you for correction. Corrections must be completed and the work resubmitted within two weeks or the grade will convert to an F. Corrections, when resubmitted, must include the original copy so that I don't have to remember what the problems were initially.

As I will be correcting these for a grade, I need to follow what you have done and how you have arrived at your answers. Therefore, it behooves you to be neat and show a relatively logical progression. This may mean you need to redo your original worksheet.

Treat Project Grading

I. *Recipe with quantity* (5 points) For example, milk 1 cup (indicate if whole, 2%, 1%, 1/2%, skim).

II. *Instructions for preparation* (5 points)

III. *Calorie breakdown* (25 points) List total number of calories contributed by each ingredient (include a notation indicating source of calorie information, i.e., text, package), serving size, and calories per serving. Please note that all numbers require a label. That is, 28 calories is not the same as 28 grams.

IV. *Nutrient breakdown for all ingredients with appropriate labels* (25 points) Include a notation indicating source of nutrient information (package, text, other reference).

V. *Show math and how you arrived at values/numbers* (15 points) (i.e., 3 cups at 100 cal/cup = 3 x 100 = 300 cal.)

VI. *Commentary* (25 points) The following rubric will be used for your commentary: Lacks commentary (0 points); Vague statement/no support for comment or commentary lacks quality (5 points); Incomplete commentary (could have said more) (10-20 points); Appropriate commentary (25 points)

You should be able to double check your answers by comparing the totals in grams to the totals in calories. (If your total calories from carbohydrates is 1200 calories, the total quantity of carbohydrates in grams should be about 300 grams [4 calories per gram]). As long as your results are within 10% of each other, your answer is probably correct. Food packagers have a habit of rounding things off to present their product in the best possible light.

Consider the definitions of legally defined terms when writing your commentary. See the following Web site for food item breakdowns: www.nal.usda.gov/fnic/foodcomp/. ■

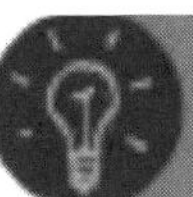

Web-Enhanced Activities

USING WEB-ENHANCED TOOLS TO TEACH CULTURAL NUTRITION PRACTICES

Teresa Johnson, Troy University School of Nursing
tjohnson@troy.edu

Most instructors find that there never seems to be enough time to cover all the topics necessary during lecture hours. We constantly seek innovative ways to engage students in the learning process, foster development of computer skills, and cover the required learning objectives of a particular nutrition lesson.

The National League for Nursing Accrediting Commission places a strong emphasis on teaching students about the diverse cultures that the nursing professional will serve. The nutrition course is an excellent and obvious vehicle in which to teach cultural diversity.

Discussion Board

All of the courses taught in the Troy University School of Nursing are Web-enhanced via Blackboard. Before the days of Web-enhanced learning, students would select a culture and complete a classroom presentation complete with handouts and visual aids. This format allowed all students to learn about many cultures but consumed much valuable classroom time. My colleague, Susie Stokes, developed the idea of having students submit their diversity reports in an online format to the Discussion Board area of Blackboard. One report is posted each week. Each student then reads the report and posts a meaningful comment within a seven-day time limit. (For larger nutrition sections, groups of 2-3 students form and complete a presentation to accommodate a 10-12 week semester.) The instructor reads the report, reads the comments, and then assigns a grade. The report earns a score and all substantive comments posted by other classmates earn a point or two. I developed a scoring rubric to guide students in preparing the report and as an assessment tool for grading. From the rubric, students can see that their report should include:

- Description of group or country
- Education level
- Leading causes of death
- Preference for Western vs alternative medicine
- Access to medical care
- Cultural/religious views and effect on health/nutrition practices
- Foods typically eaten
- Positive/negative consequences of diet

A sample report is also posted in the Discussion Board area for students to read. (You can visit www.aw-bc.com/greatideas to see a sample student report and the complete scoring rubric.)

Benefits

This approach to teaching cultural diversity is excellent in that all students benefit from the work of others in the classroom, computer skills are encouraged, opportunity to utilize writing skills is offered, collaboration is encouraged, and valuable classroom time is saved. Cultural diversity instruction is offered in this same format for the online nutrition courses and works very well. The online population is scattered over a large region, but students are able to collaborate and benefit from the collective class efforts. ■

ENGAGING STUDENTS ON THE WEB AND IN THE CLASSROOM

Allison Miner, Prince George's Community College
aminer@pgcc.edu

I use a lot of incentives to help my students become more engaged in the subject of nutrition and science and to increase their retention of the material.

continued on page 142

Engaging Students on the Web and in the Classroom
continued from page 141

Extra Credit Online

In my online course, I have "surprise" extra points given throughout the entire semester. Because students never know when these points will be available, they are more alert and I get much more participation and attendance. For instance, I pose extra credit questions on the Announcements page once per week or more. These extra credit questions have to do with the topic we are covering and pop up randomly. (This is achieved through a feature of Blackboard.) I try and focus on questions not covered in the textbook so it forces students to think about facets of nutrition other than what is traditionally covered. The first student to correctly answer the question by posting to the Discussion Board gets the extra credit. Students learn quickly that I don't take answers that are merely copied from other sources or those that don't specifically answer the question that I pose. Here are some examples of questions I have used:

- Little Johnny has been diagnosed with lead poisoning. Is this a problem? Which micronutrients are involved?
- Little Johnny has hypercarotenemia. What is it? Is it dangerous?
- Rat poison contains a substance that works against one of the micronutrients. What is that micronutrient and how does rat poison work?
- What are these compounds and which of the micronutrients form a part of their structure: ATP, HCl, Acetyl CoA, Hydroxyapatite, Hemoglobin?
- What is hypokalemia and why does it occur?
- Lactaid milk tastes sweeter than regular milk. Why?
- As you know, the number of trans fatty acids in various food products will be required on food labels beginning in 2006. Until then, how can consumers (using the Nutrition Facts Food Label) determine if a food products contains trans fatty acids?

Although these don't amount to a significant number of points, students log on several times per day to check for messages from me and extra credit opportunities. This keeps the course exciting and challenging.

Oral Presentations in the Classroom

For my face-to-face courses, everyone must complete an oral presentation on a nutrition topic that the student and I agree upon. However, all students must participate in that presentation. It is a requirement that students ask questions of the speaker and that the speaker be prepared to answer and know how to respond. The students giving the presentation must know more than what they present and this forces them to become much more familiar with their topic. It also increases students' confidence when they can answer intelligently about a topic they have researched. The student audience is also tasked to ask intelligent questions about the topic, so they must pay attention to the speaker and think beyond what has been presented. I am always amazed and pleased when our department invites the entire campus to hear various scientific presentations given by invited professionals and my students are the ones asking all the questions (I don't require that they do this). They have learned to think beyond the presentation and that asking questions is an important feature of learning. ■

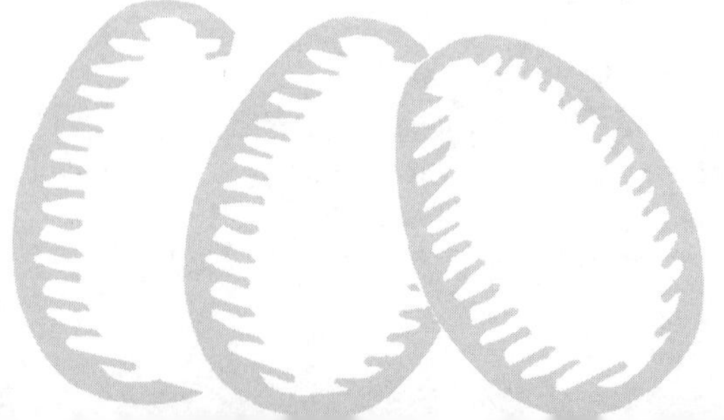